Niki Guinn-Rogers
Email: nikiguinnrogers@gmail.com

TgosketchPress
Chicago, Illinois
www.tgosketch.com

I'd like to thank my husband, Vitto, who has been my
biggest support during this project. To my children Aiden, Hailee & Amiaya, who never asked
questions, just simply loved. To my family and friends whose unwavering support and prayers
have helped along the way. I dedicate this book to my mom who showed me how to fight until
the end. And to the countless boys & girls whose parents get sick- always remember...
Kids Fight Too!

Niki Guinn-Rogers

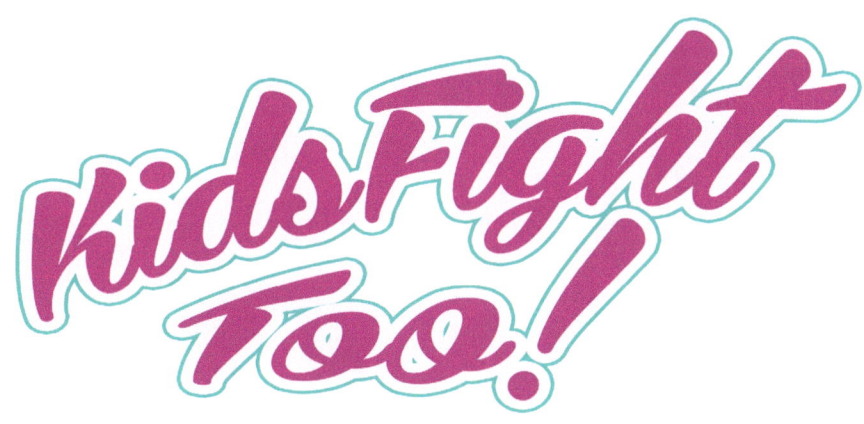

The sun shined brightly through Brynn Jean's window. The bright beams warmed her face and woke her with a smile. She opened her eyes and suddenly realized it was not an ordinary day, it was her birthday!

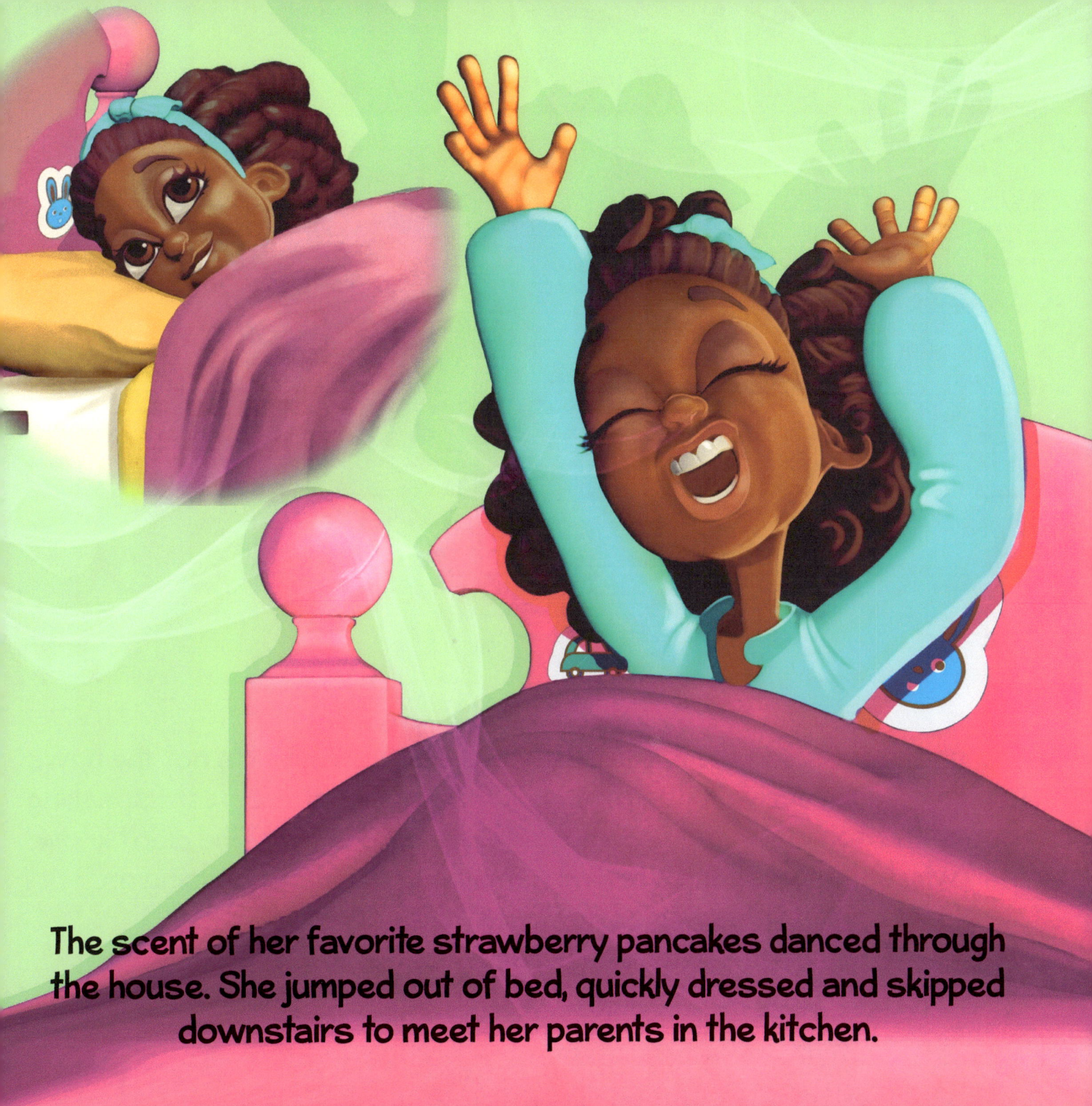

The scent of her favorite strawberry pancakes danced through the house. She jumped out of bed, quickly dressed and skipped downstairs to meet her parents in the kitchen.

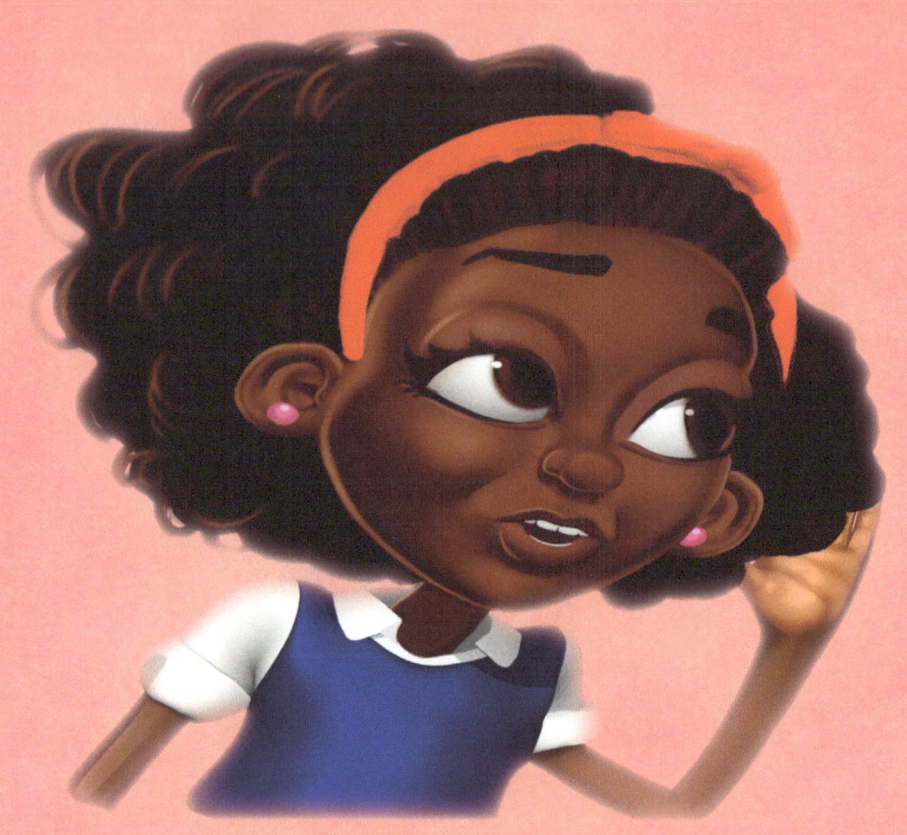

As she approached them, she overheard her mom say, "It's not the news I'd expected to receive today." Brynn didn't know what they were speaking about and something between her parents felt different. She didn't know why but she just had a feeling something unusual was going on. Determined not to let their secrecy ruin her special day, she barged into the kitchen proudly.

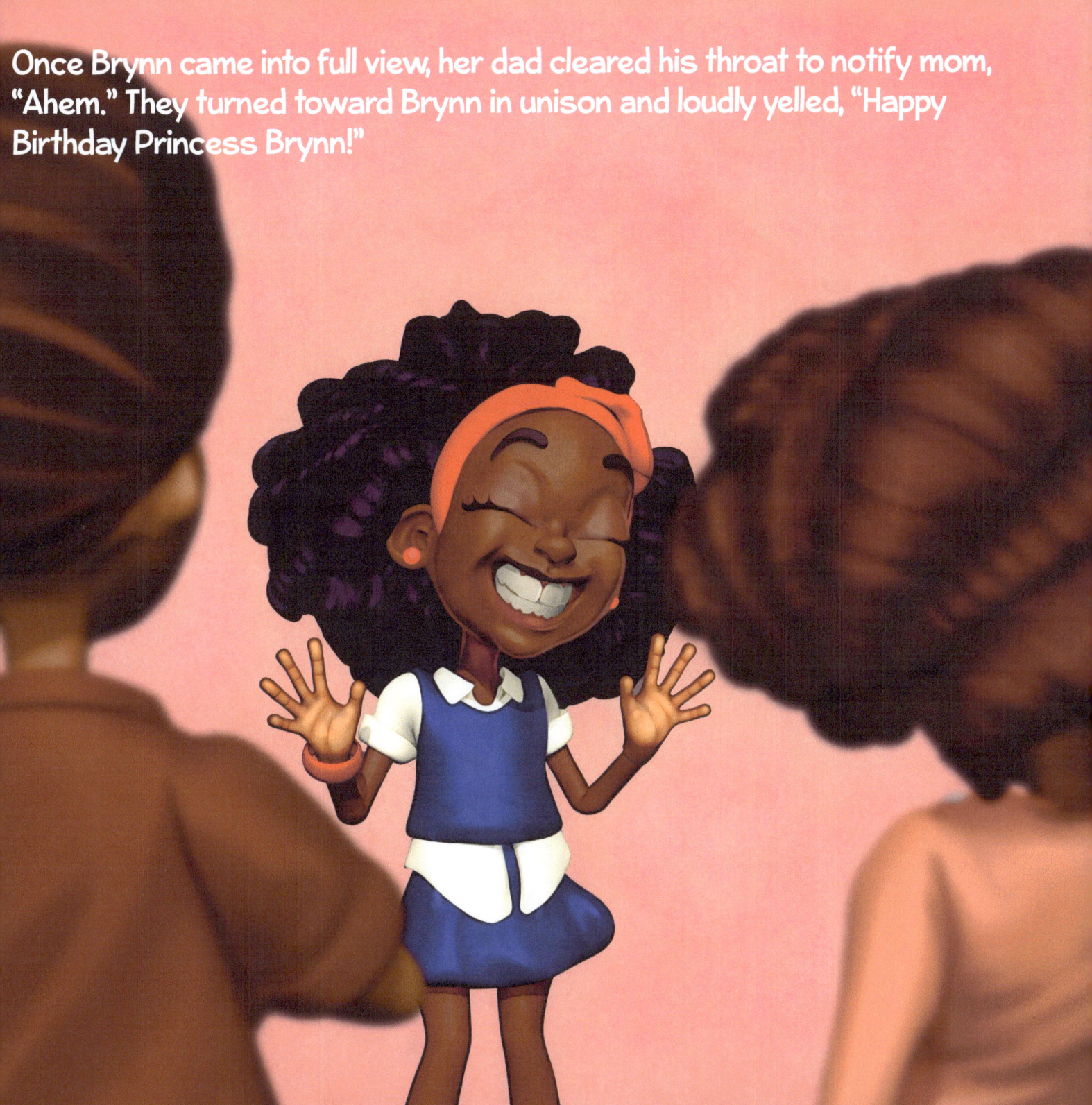

Once Brynn came into full view, her dad cleared his throat to notify mom, "Ahem." They turned toward Brynn in unison and loudly yelled, "Happy Birthday Princess Brynn!"

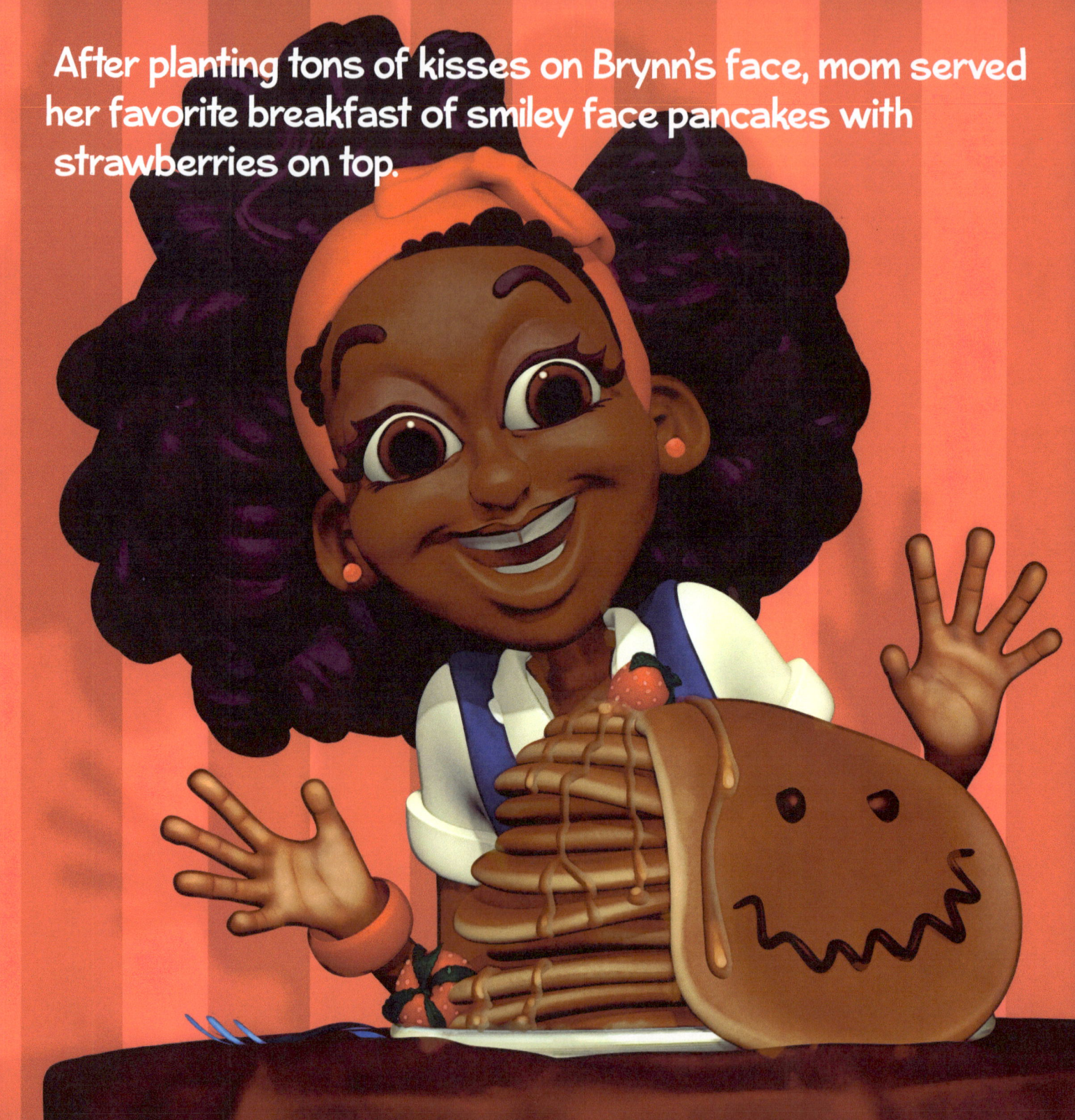

After planting tons of kisses on Brynn's face, mom served her favorite breakfast of smiley face pancakes with strawberries on top.

"You'd better hurry honey, so you won't miss your bus," mom said. "I promise to have your birthday cupcakes baked, decorated and delivered just in time for lunch," mom said. As she gathered her backpack to head to the bus, the worried look on her parent's faces did not go unnoticed.

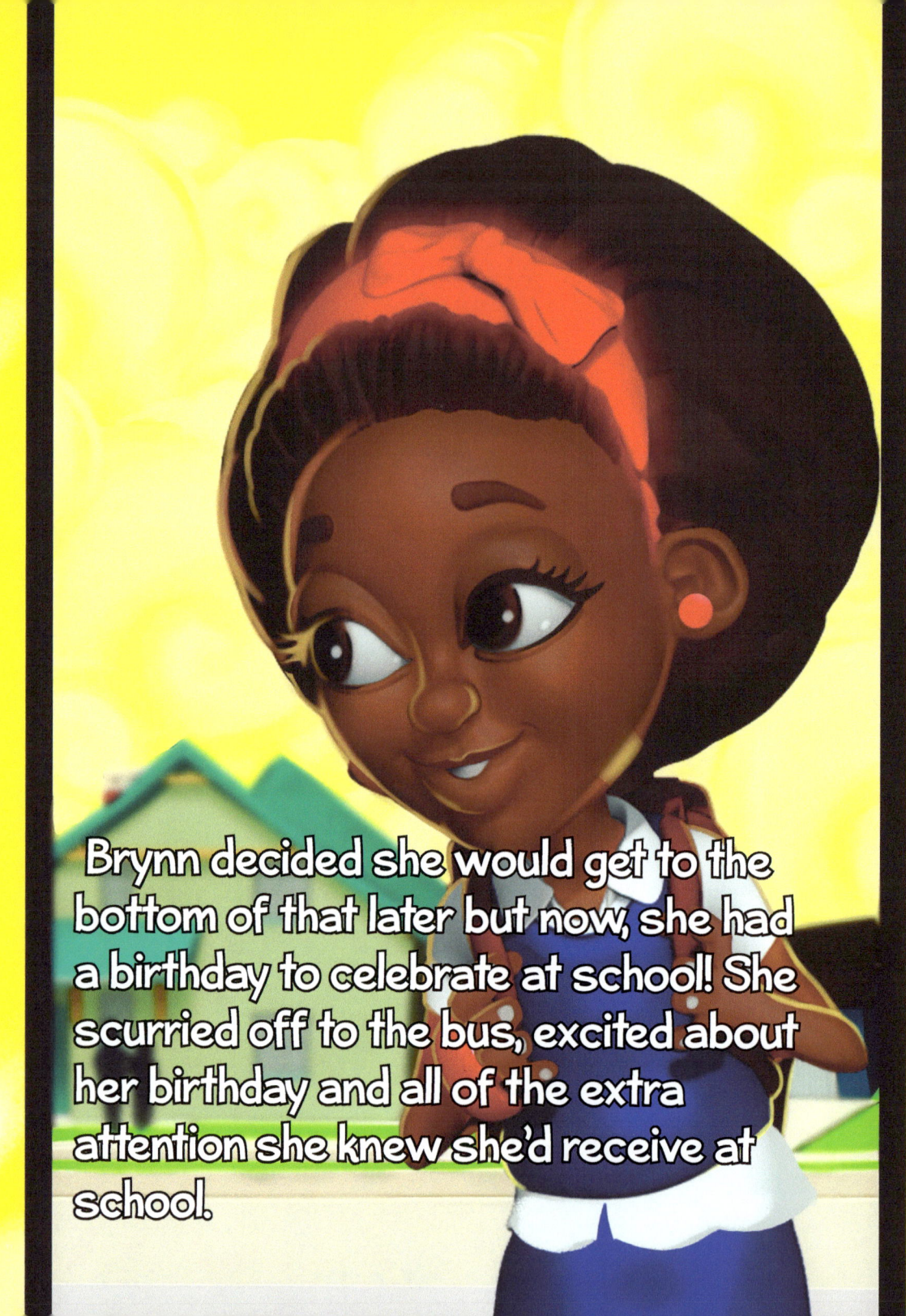

Brynn decided she would get to the bottom of that later but now, she had a birthday to celebrate at school! She scurried off to the bus, excited about her birthday and all of the extra attention she knew she'd receive at school.

The ride to school seemed to take forever. This was the last week of school before summer break and the kids seated near her were all excitedly discussing their plans for the summer. As the students chatted loudly, all Brynn could think about was the big birthday party she and her mom would soon be planning. Brynn could hardly wait.

Once at school, Brynn loved all the extra special attention she was receiving. She was able to be line leader for the day and had a received a collection of handmade cards from her classmates. Her birthday was off to a great start.

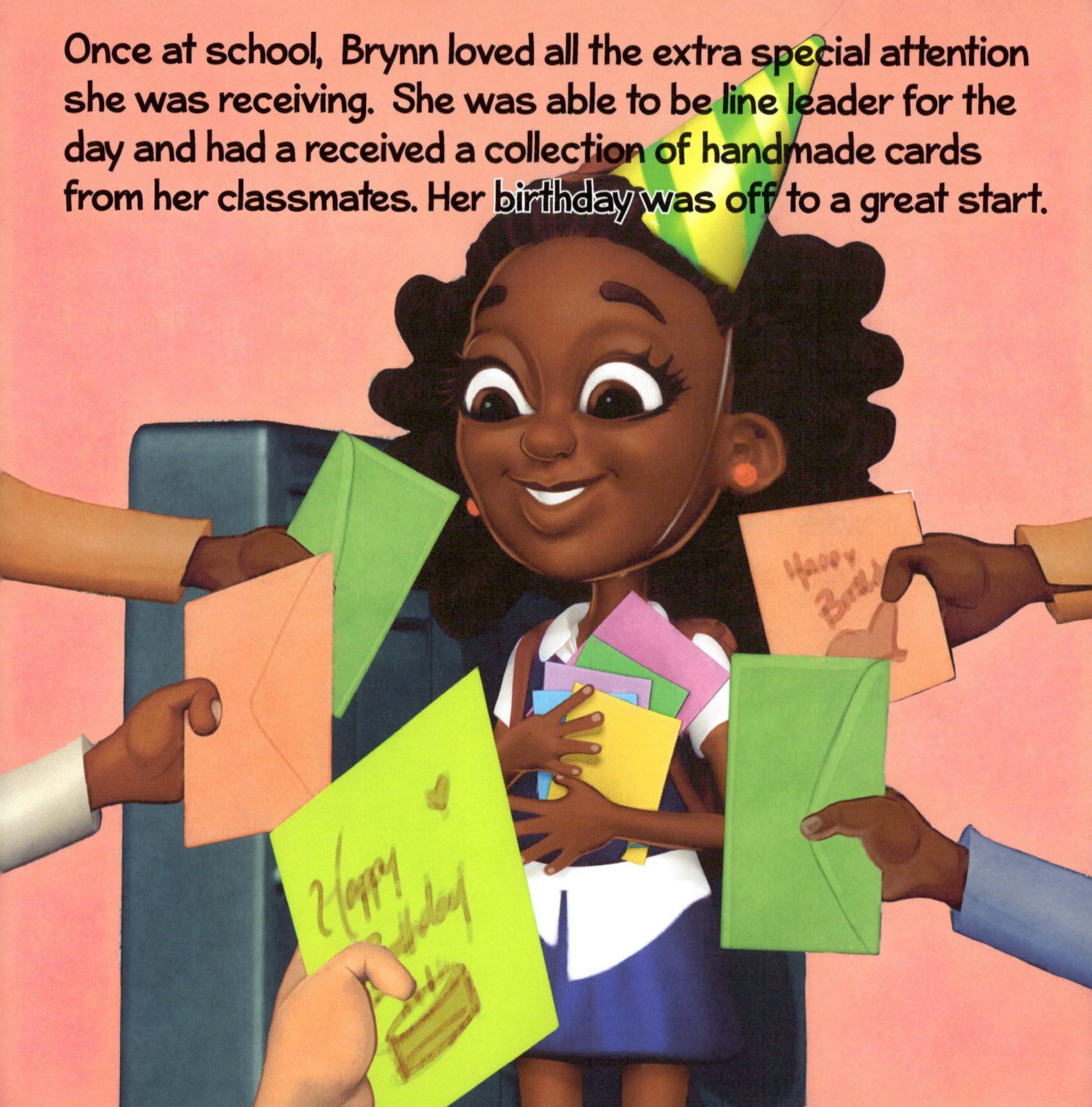

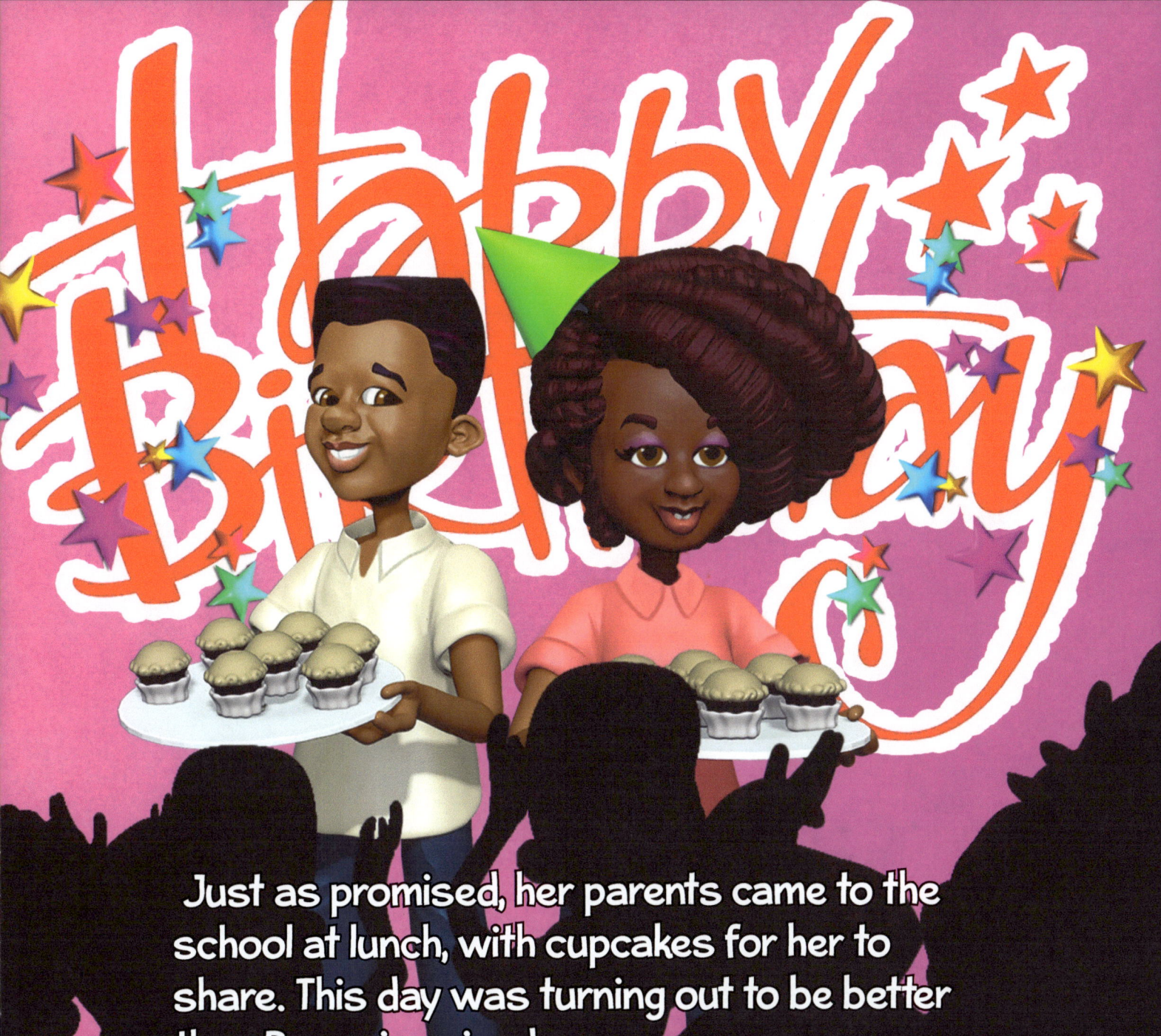

Just as promised, her parents came to the school at lunch, with cupcakes for her to share. This day was turning out to be better than Brynn imagined.

That night, as mom came to tuck her in and to read her nightly story, there was still no mention of the party. Brynn was so exhausted that she fell fast asleep before the story was complete.

Brynn's parents told her that there'd been a change in plans for the upcoming week. That would be the first week of summer break and it was her party week so Brynn was immediately all ears for the new details.

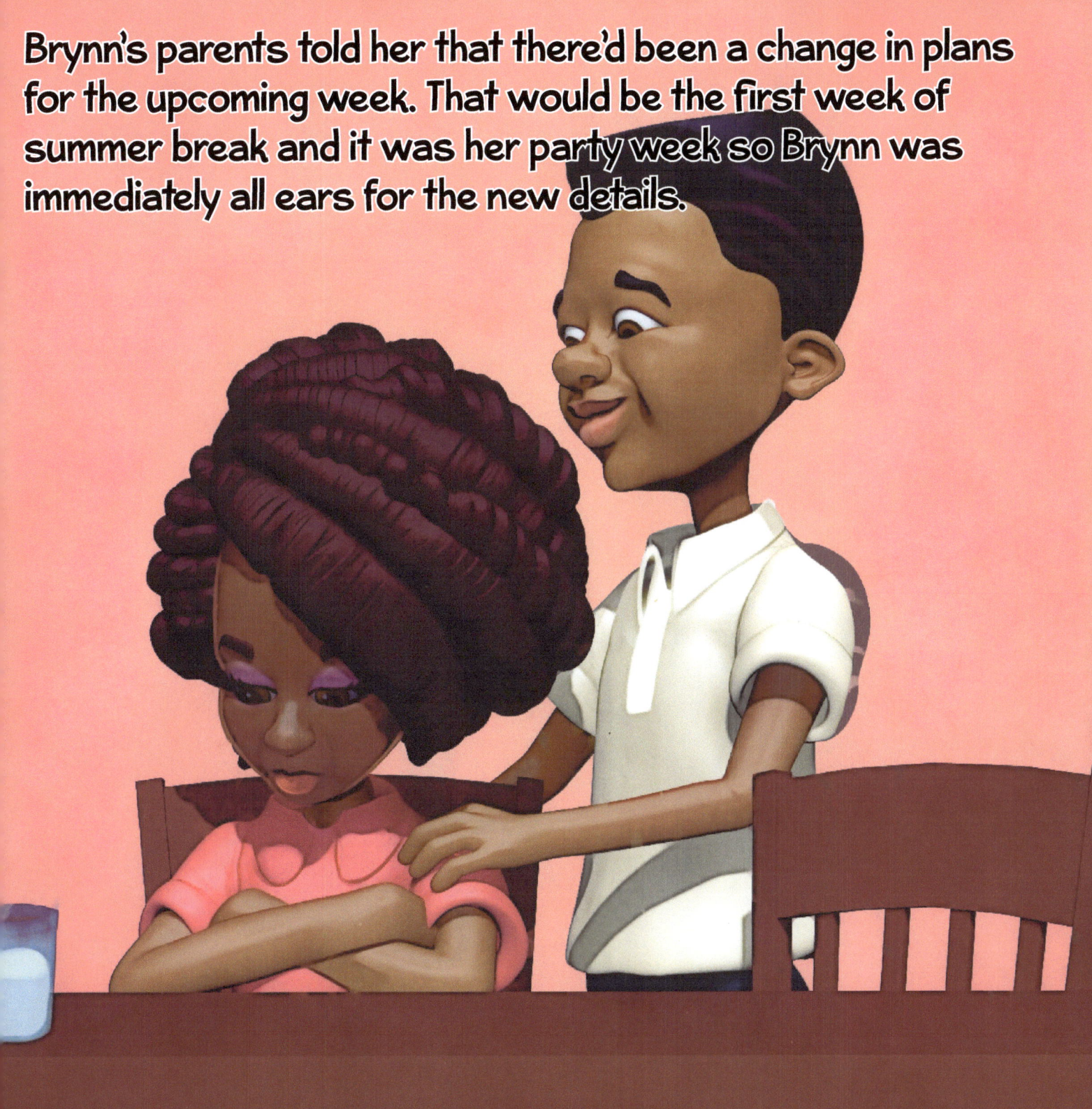

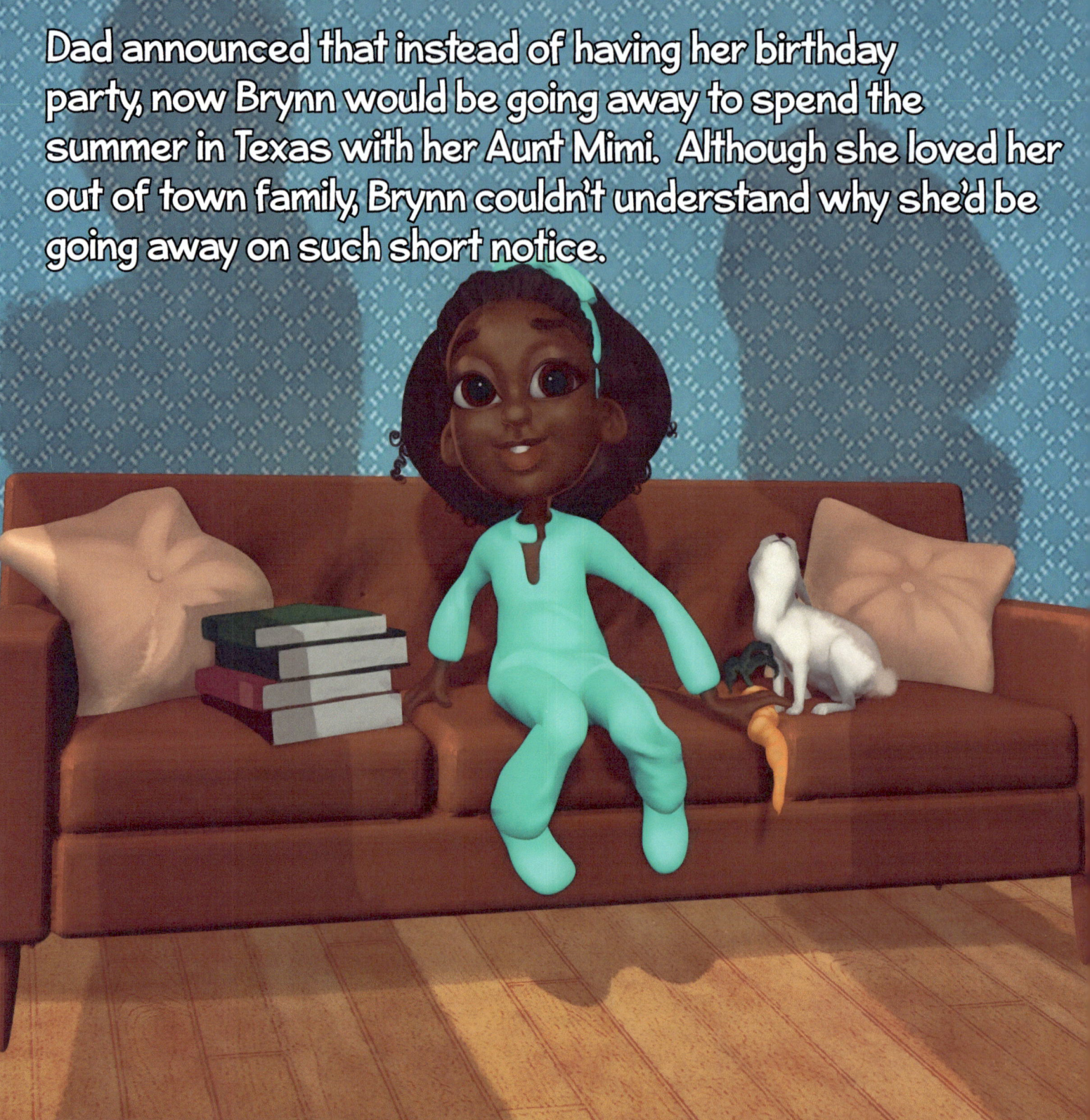

Dad announced that instead of having her birthday party, now Brynn would be going away to spend the summer in Texas with her Aunt Mimi. Although she loved her out of town family, Brynn couldn't understand why she'd be going away on such short notice.

Dad explained that mom had recently been diagnosed with an illness that would require her to have surgery, take medicine and get plenty of rest in order to get better.

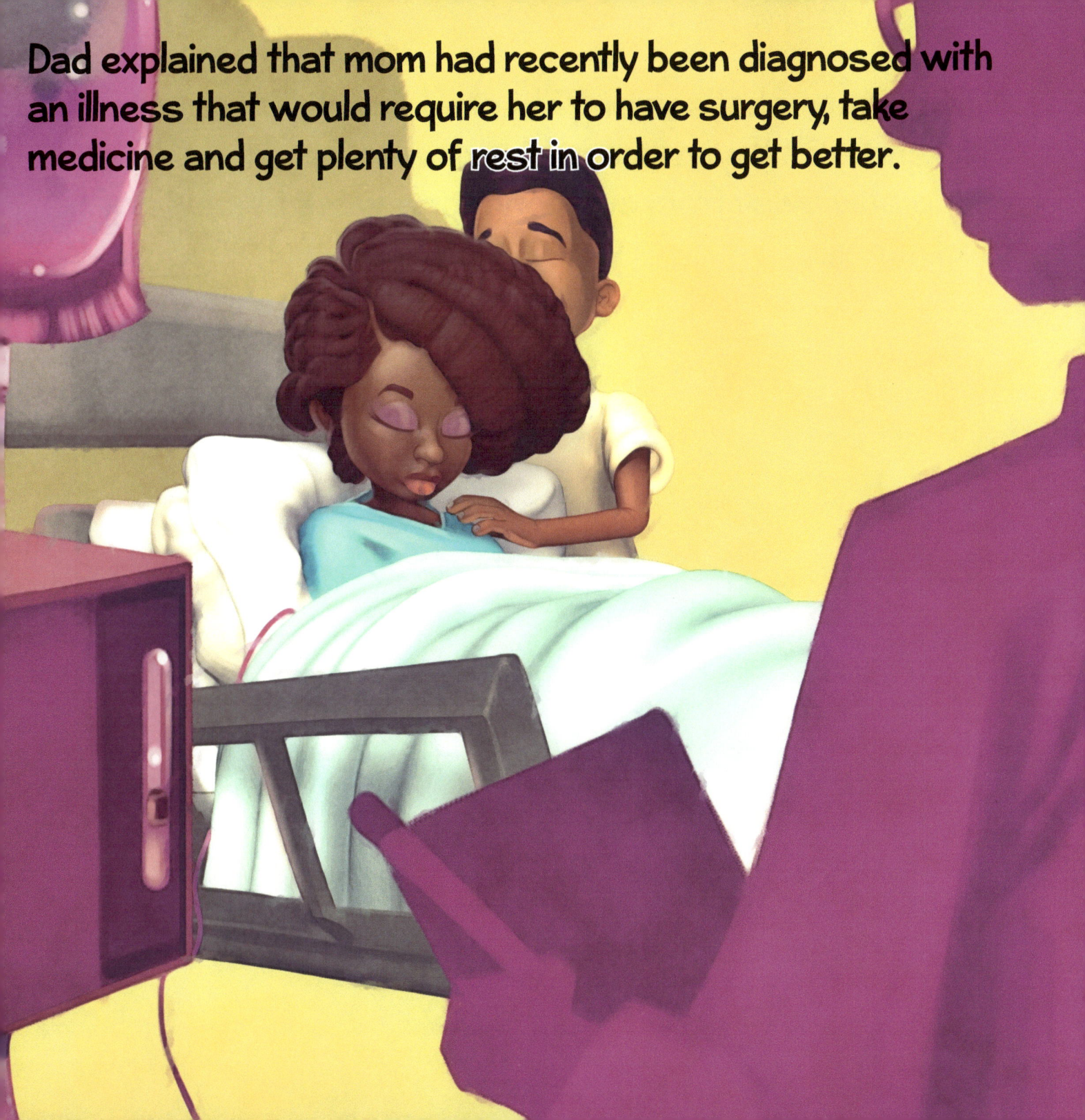

"Oh mommy, what's wrong?" Asked Brynn. "Do you have Chickenpox?" Brynn remembered when her friend, Aiden had to stay away from everyone for a week because of his Chickenpox.

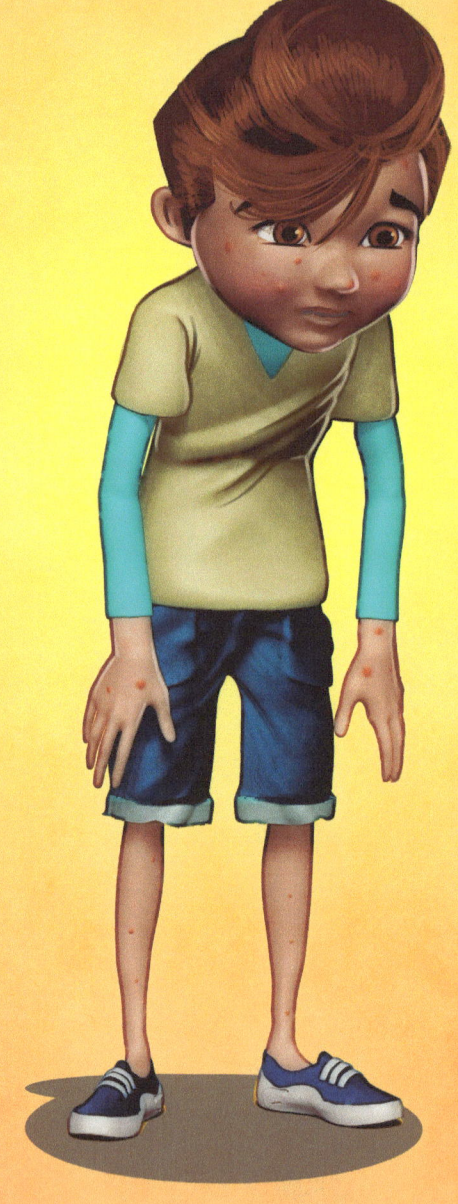

"I'm afraid it's a bit more serious than that," dad explained. "Brynn, Mom was recently diagnosed with breast cancer," said dad. "What is breast cancer?" Brynn asked. She had no idea what it was but could tell it wasn't good from the way her parents had been acting lately.

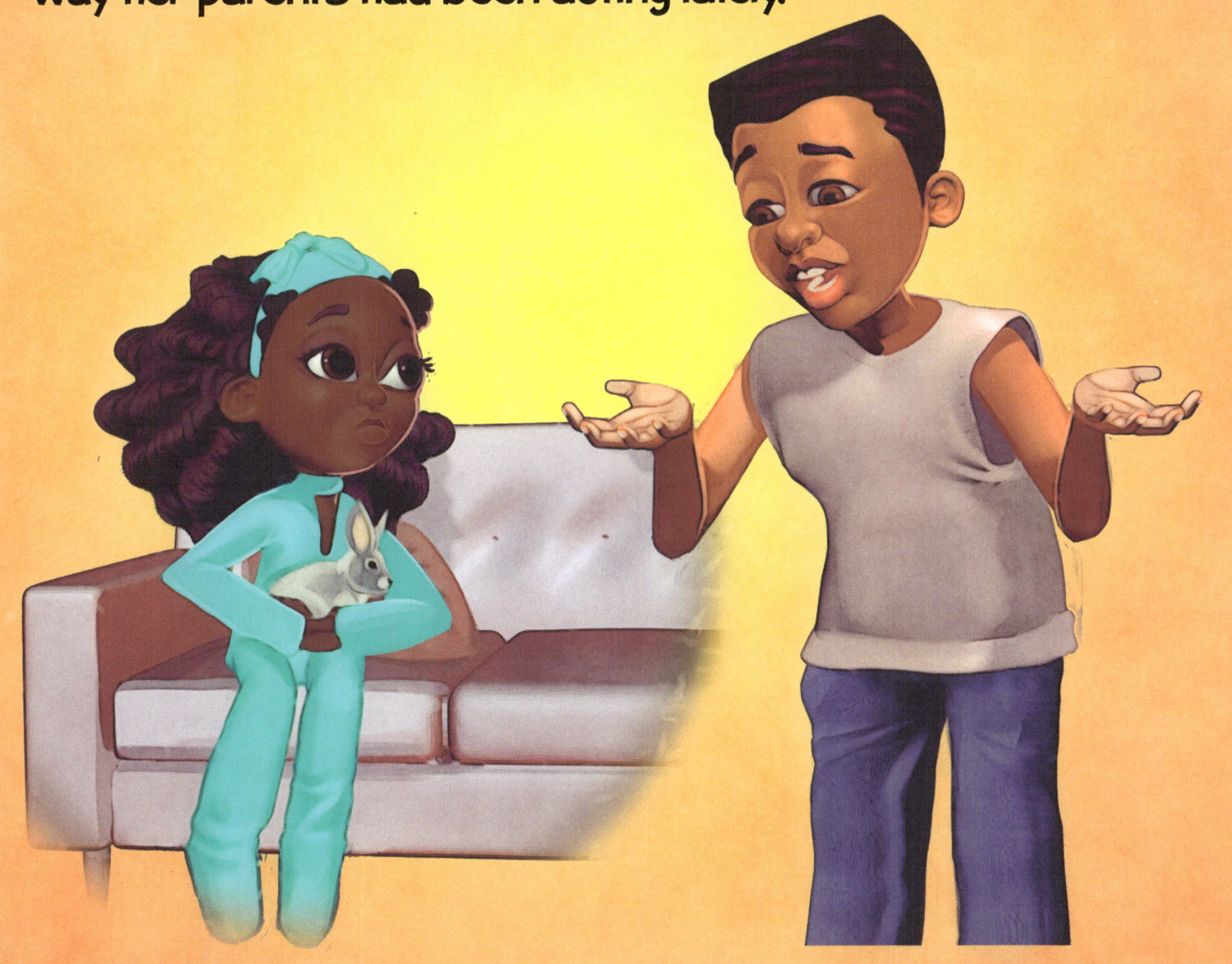

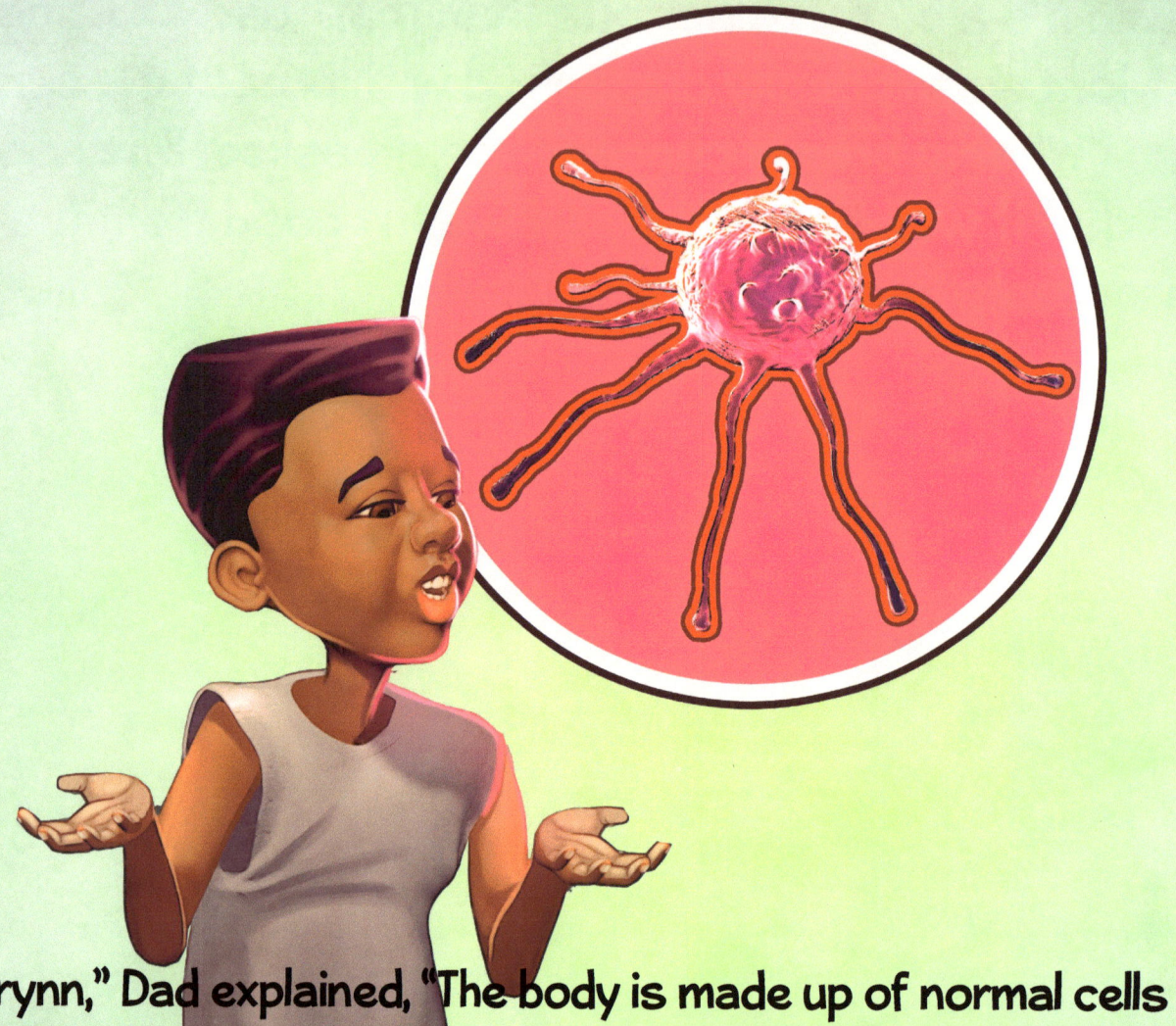

"Brynn," Dad explained, "The body is made up of normal cells to help it function. Cancer develops when abnormal cells begin to take over the normal cells. When the bad cells aren't controlled they make a person very sick." "Well how can we get rid of the bad cells Brynn asked?" "There were several ways to treat the cancer and to destroy the bad cells. In mom's case, the doctors feel that since her cancer was found early, they can remove the cancer through surgery and through giving mom a strong medicine called Chemotherapy, (Chemo for short).

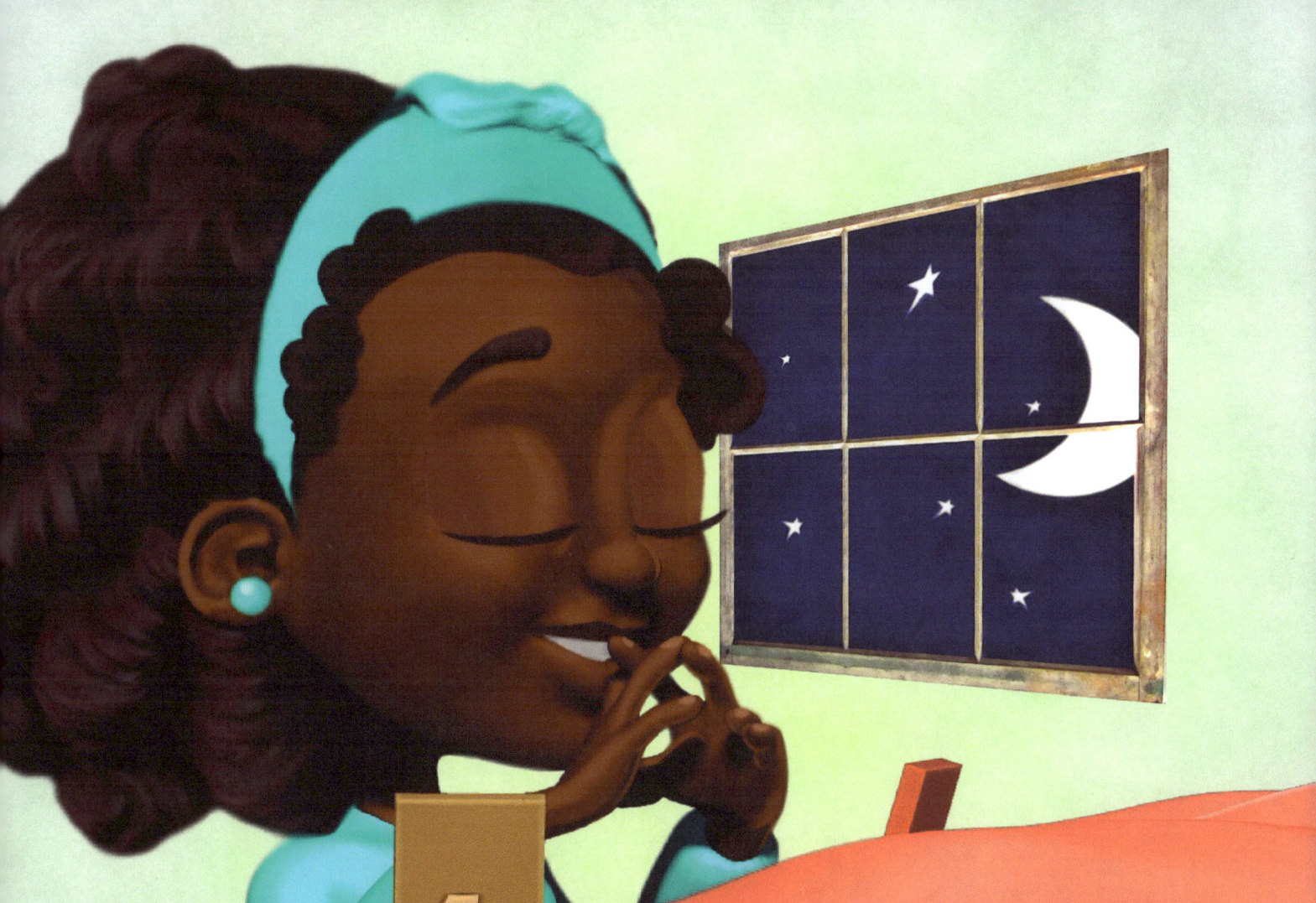

That night, Brynn felt afraid and worried for her mom. She felt sad because she really didn't understand how cancer worked and without knowing how it worked, she wasn't able to help her mom get better. During her prayers, she asked God to protect mommy, to allow the medicine to work and to take the cancer away.

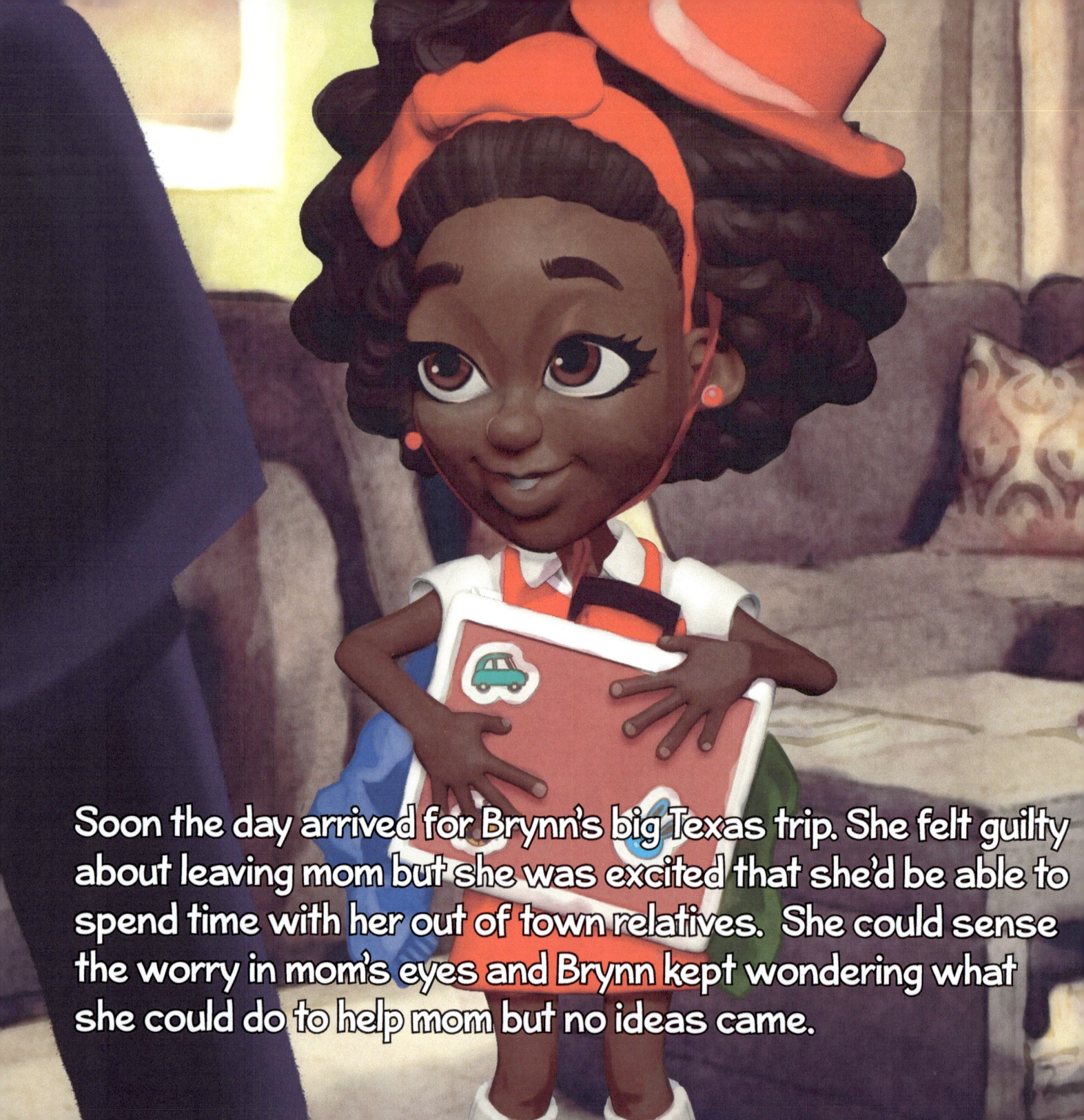

Soon the day arrived for Brynn's big Texas trip. She felt guilty about leaving mom but she was excited that she'd be able to spend time with her out of town relatives. She could sense the worry in mom's eyes and Brynn kept wondering what she could do to help mom but no ideas came.

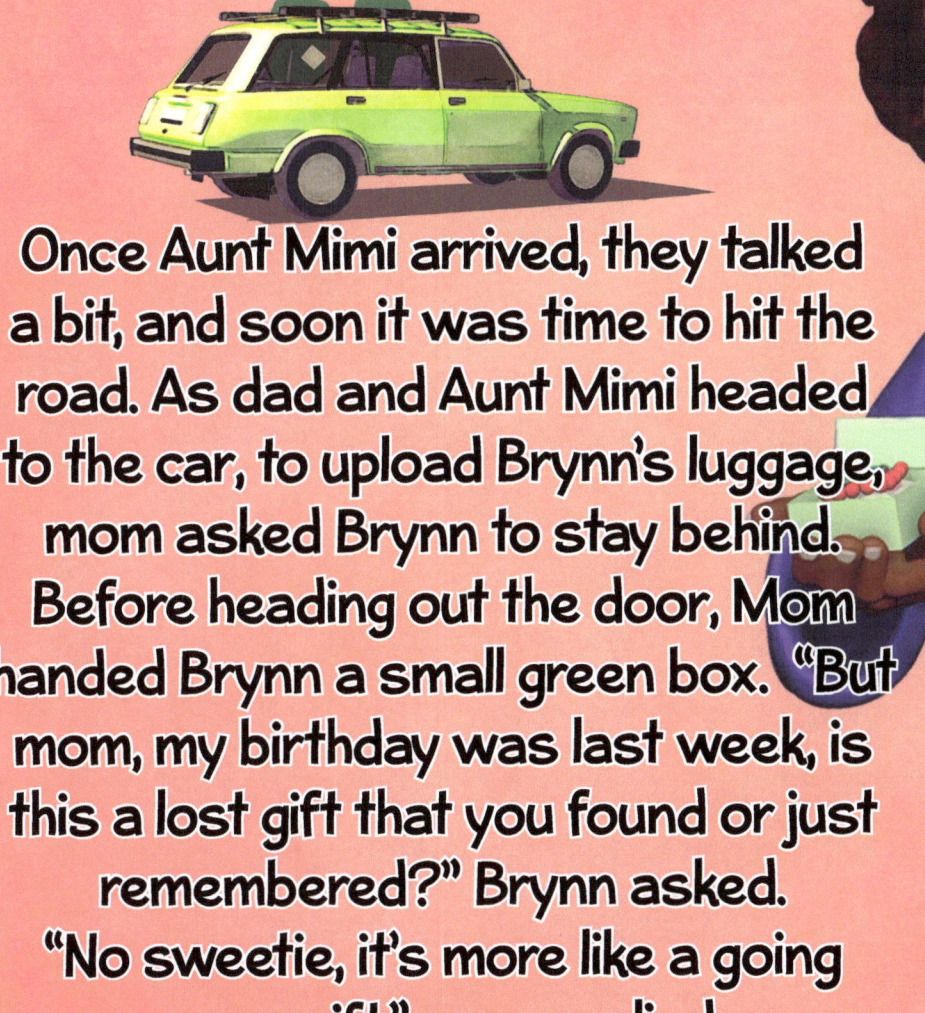

Once Aunt Mimi arrived, they talked a bit, and soon it was time to hit the road. As dad and Aunt Mimi headed to the car, to upload Brynn's luggage, mom asked Brynn to stay behind. Before heading out the door, Mom handed Brynn a small green box. "But mom, my birthday was last week, is this a lost gift that you found or just remembered?" Brynn asked. "No sweetie, it's more like a going away gift," mom replied.

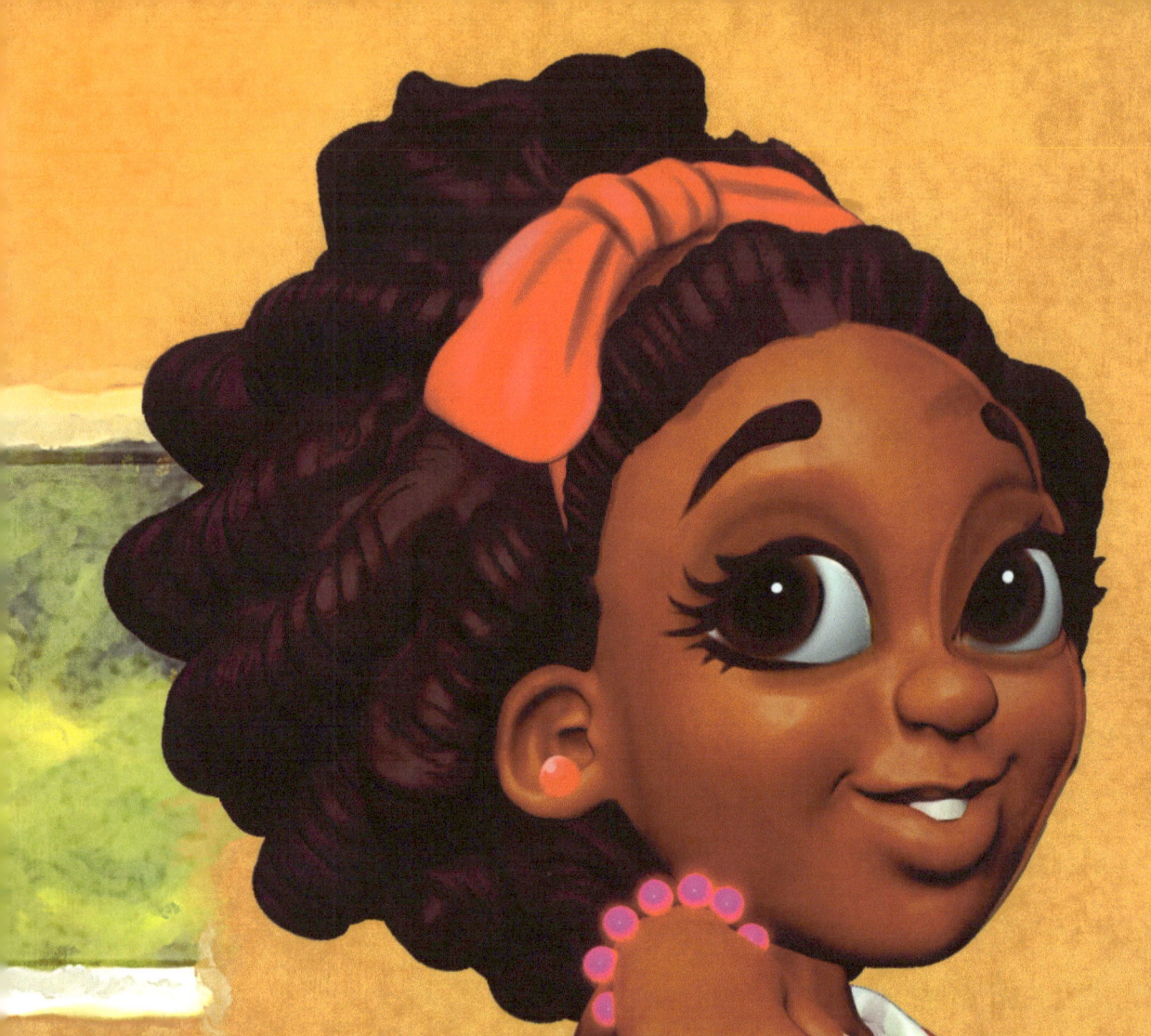

When Brynn opened the box she found an adorable pink bracelet with black block letters that read, "Kids Fight Too." "The bracelet is pink because pink is the recognized color for breast cancer Brynn, and I want you to know that during our separation, I know you'll be worried about me.

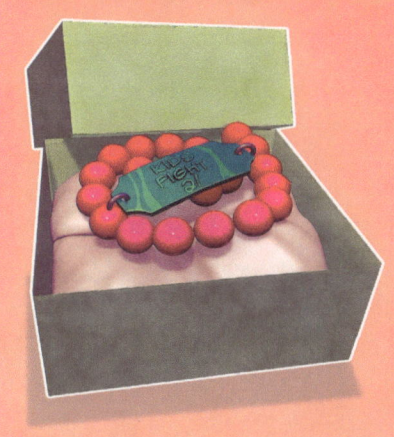

As you wear this bracelet, let it remind you that "Kids Fight Too." "Kids fight through their thoughts, and their prayers. So even though you'll be in Texas, just know that you are still supporting me and that will help me through," mom said. Brynn slid the bracelet over her wrist she noticed that her mom wore one too. She seemed to instantly feel better as she wore it. She gave her parents big hugs and was off to Texas.

Brynn spent the summer in Texas and had a blast during that time. She enjoyed playing with her cousins, learning new games, eating more candy and junk food than her parents normally allowed and she especially liked how Aunt Mimi let her stay up extra late most nights.

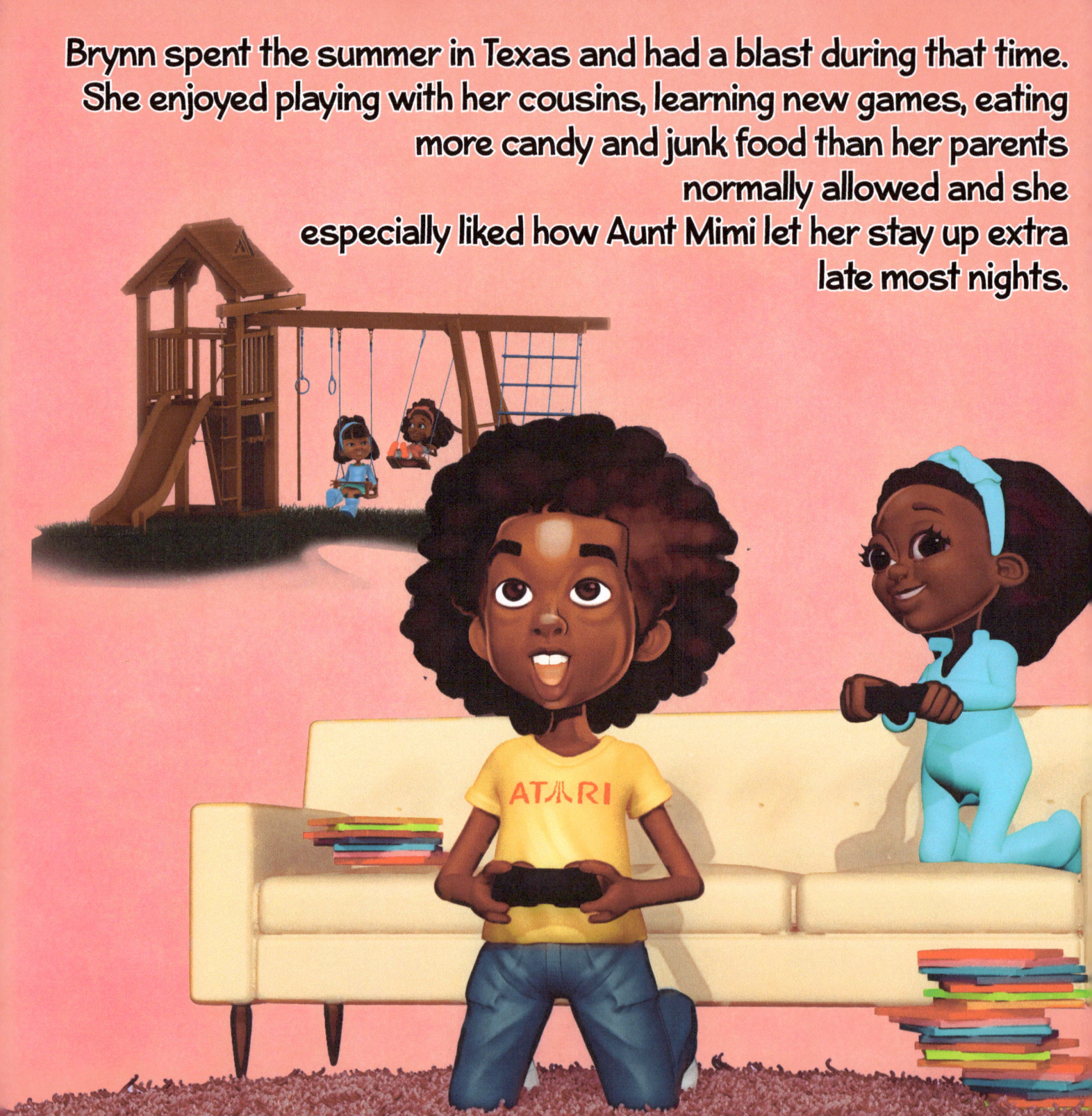

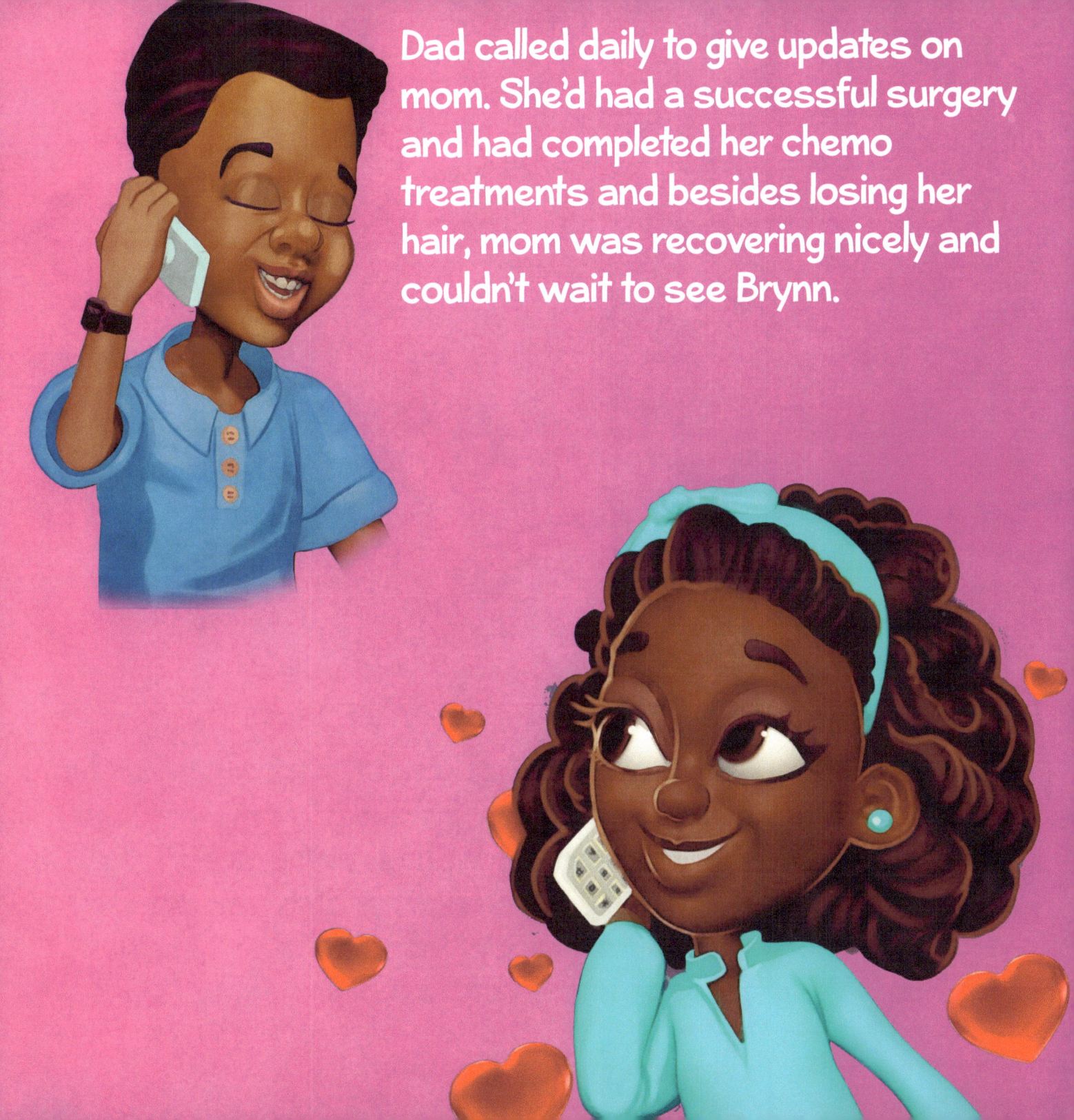

Dad called daily to give updates on mom. She'd had a successful surgery and had completed her chemo treatments and besides losing her hair, mom was recovering nicely and couldn't wait to see Brynn.

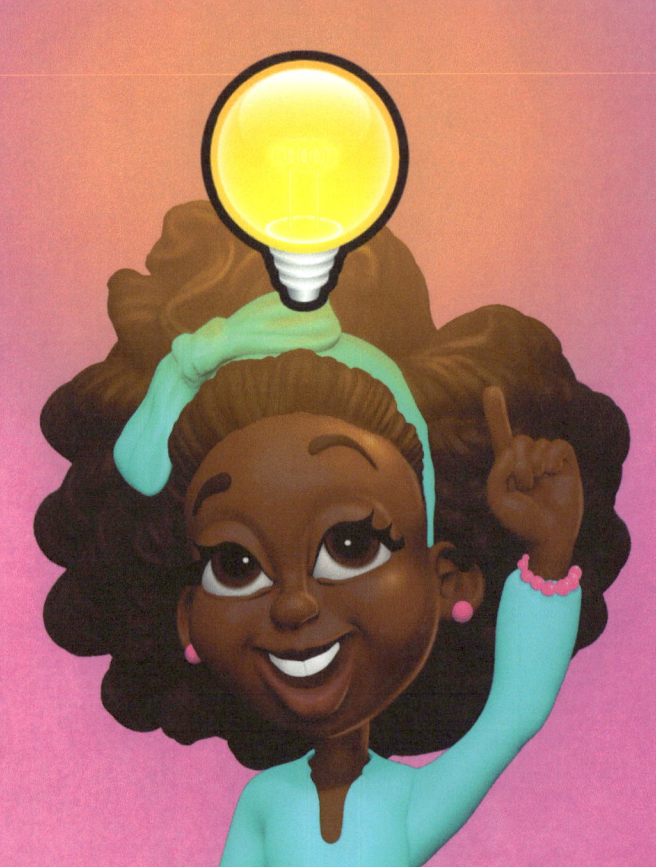

Even with the regular updates, Brynn was still worried about mom. She couldn't stop thinking of what she could do to make things better. One day, as she looked down at her pink bracelet, she had a bright idea. Brynn was going to design her own support shirt with the same saying as the bracelet mom had given her. "Aunt Mimi, can you take me to the craft store?" Brynn asked. "Sure," her aunt replied.

Once at the store, Brynn was eager to gather materials she needed for her project. She picked up a pink shirt, fabric paint, paint brushes and scissors. When they returned home, Brynn went to work on her shirt creation project.

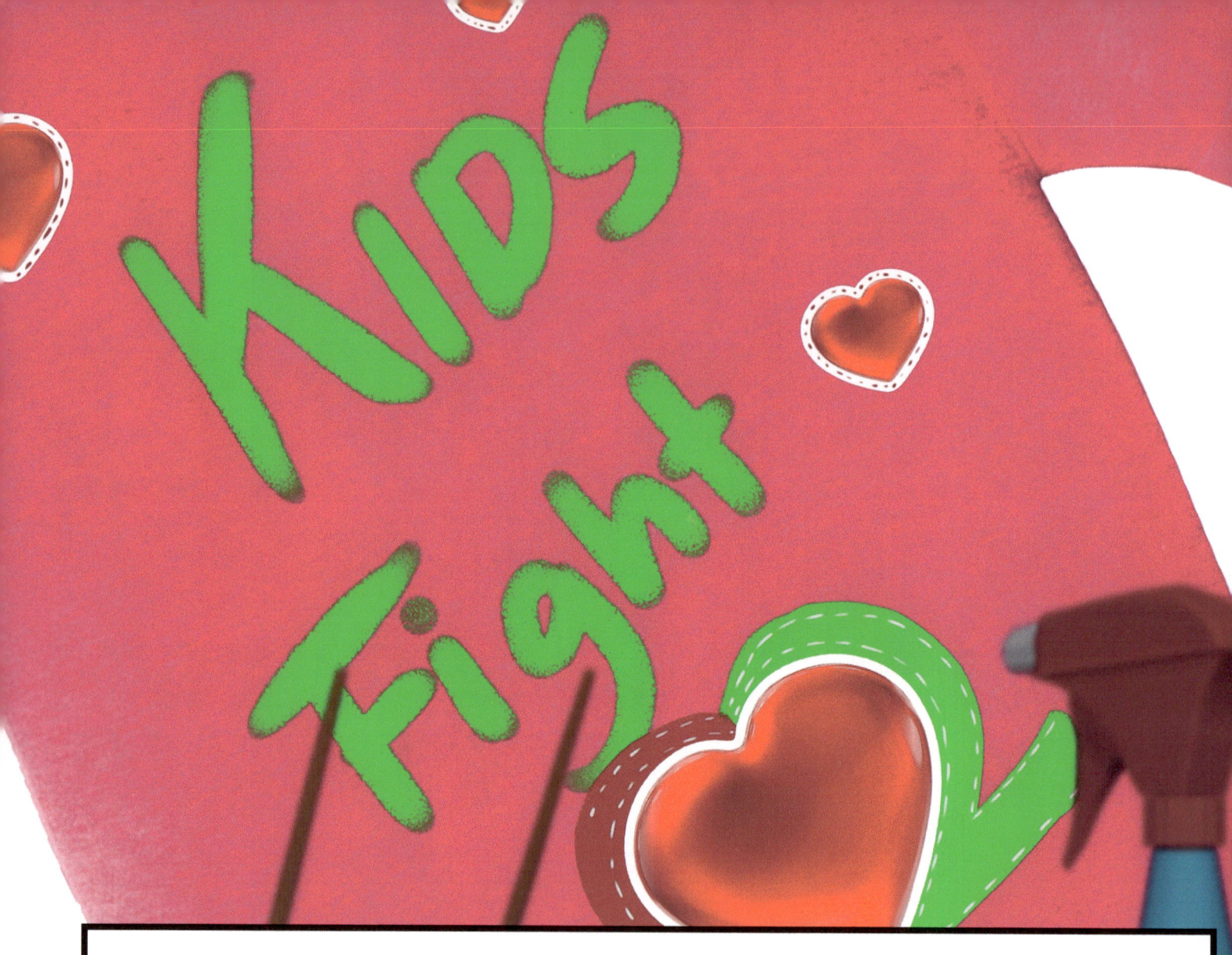

She quickly laid out the materials and went to work on her design. She laid the pink shirt out and used rainbow colors to write Kids Fight 2. She even etched the cancer awareness ribbon onto her shirt and cut fancy slits at the bottom.

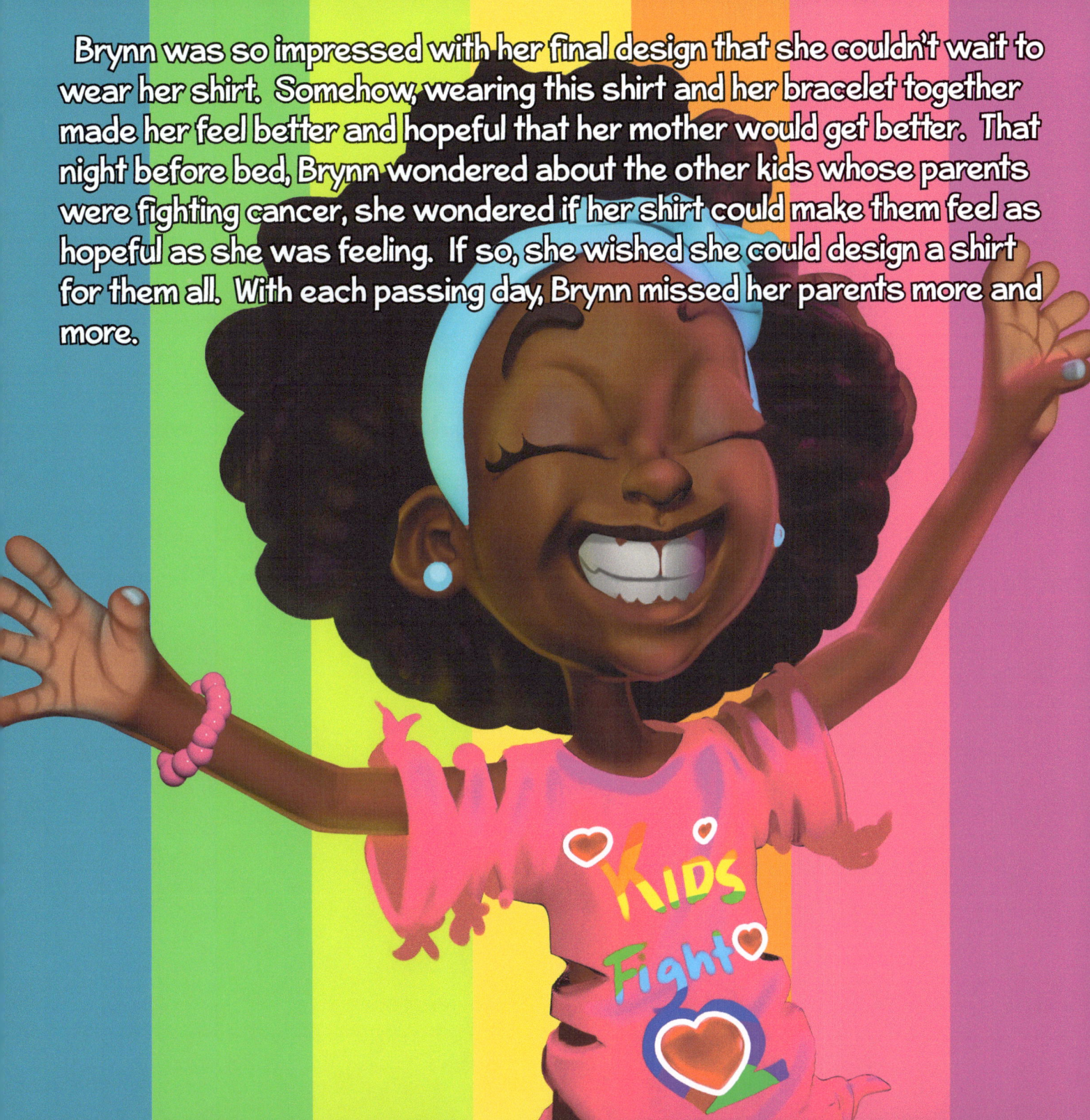

Brynn was so impressed with her final design that she couldn't wait to wear her shirt. Somehow, wearing this shirt and her bracelet together made her feel better and hopeful that her mother would get better. That night before bed, Brynn wondered about the other kids whose parents were fighting cancer, she wondered if her shirt could make them feel as hopeful as she was feeling. If so, she wished she could design a shirt for them all. With each passing day, Brynn missed her parents more and more.

Her Texas time soon came to an end and it was time to return home. The ride home seemed to have taken much longer than the ride to Texas. Brynn was both excited and nervous to see her mom. She'd heard that cancer patients sometimes looked different so she felt afraid and unsure of what to expect once they arrived home.

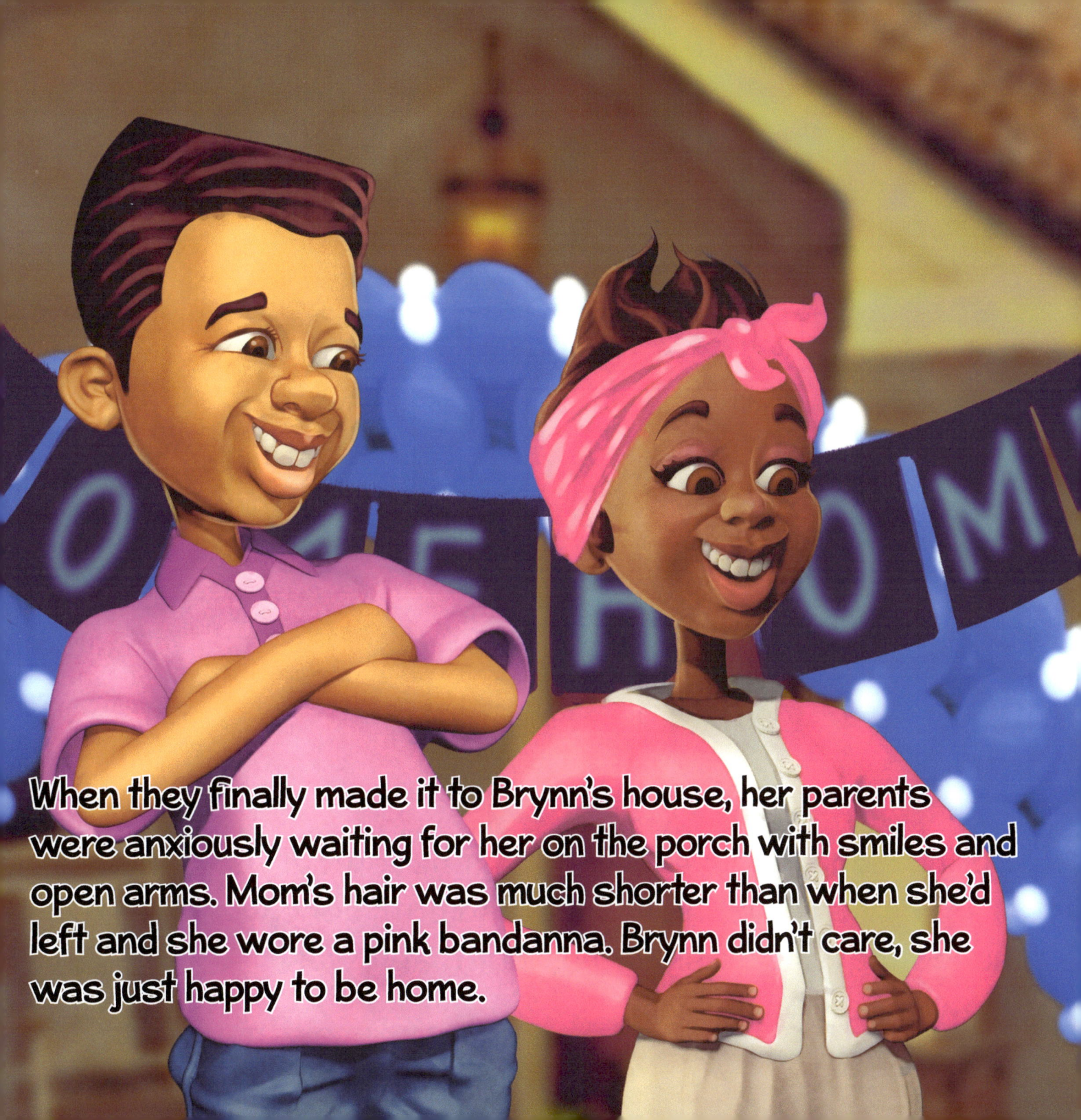

When they finally made it to Brynn's house, her parents were anxiously waiting for her on the porch with smiles and open arms. Mom's hair was much shorter than when she'd left and she wore a pink bandanna. Brynn didn't care, she was just happy to be home.

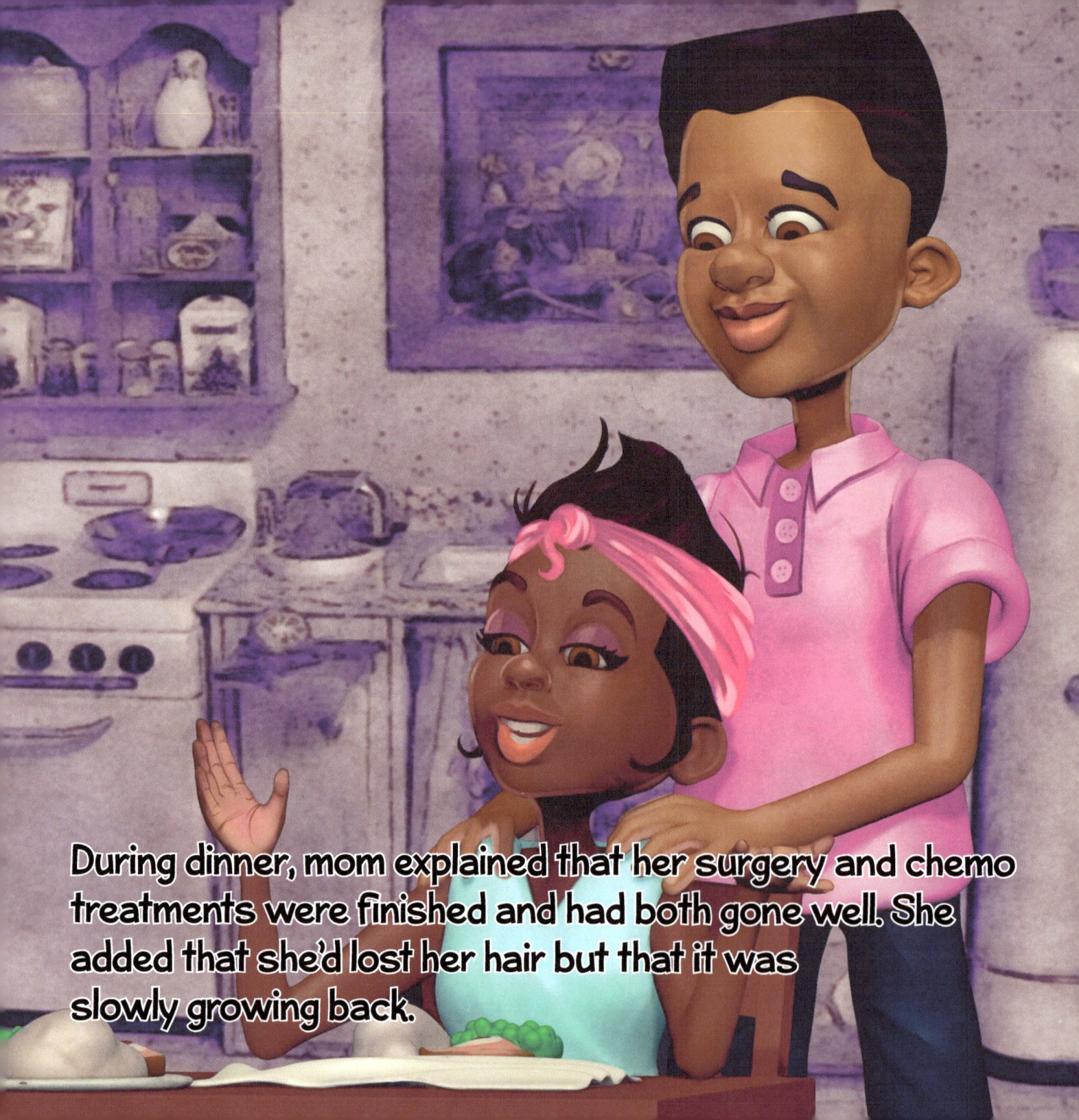

During dinner, mom explained that her surgery and chemo treatments were finished and had both gone well. She added that she'd lost her hair but that it was slowly growing back.

Her doctor wanted her to take it easy because she needed to let her body rest and heal. Mom said she was glad that Brynn was home and that she knew with Brynn's help, she'd get stronger each day.

Brynn got excited and asked mom if her breast cancer was all gone. Her parents explained that they wouldn't know anything until mom had her final doctor's follow up visit and that they'd go to that appointment together as a family.

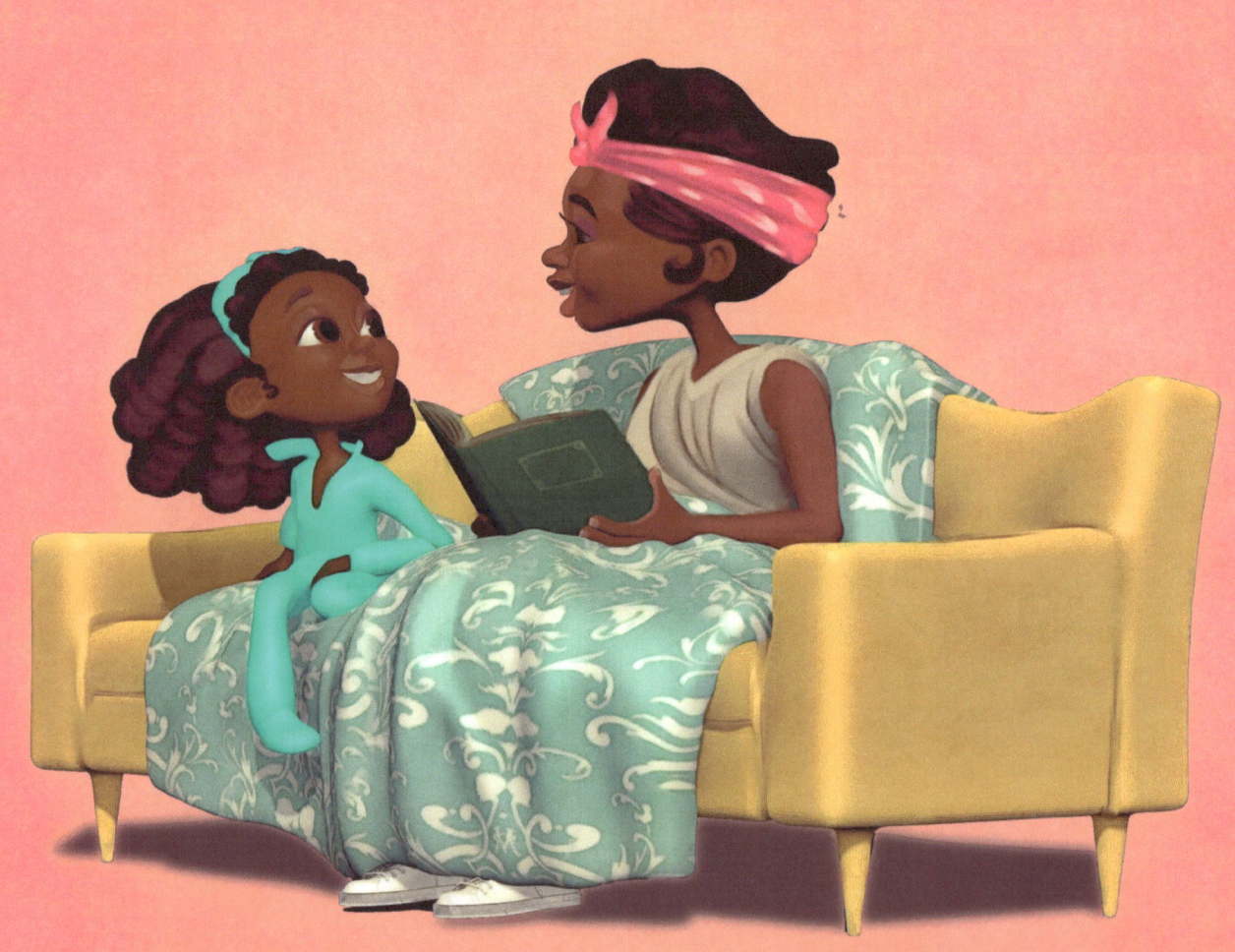

The family settled back into their normal routine, and mom seemed to be well on her way to recovery. The time quickly came for mom's big appointment. This was an important appointment because mom would find out the status of her cancer treatment. The entire family would be going to this appointment to support mom.

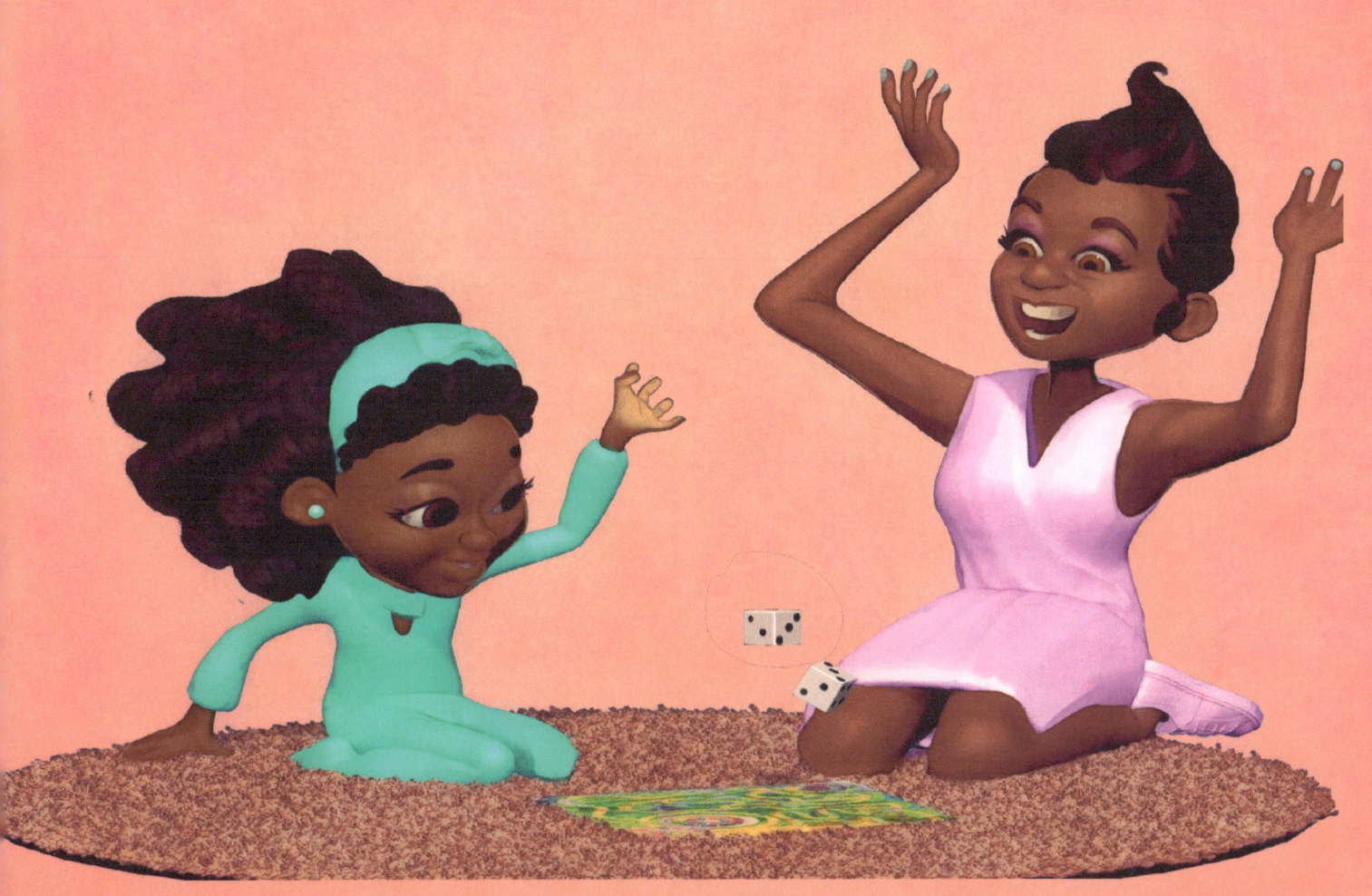

On the big appointment day, Brynn wore her Kids Fight 2 shirt & bracelet. She felt she needed the happiness and hopeful feelings that came with wearing them.

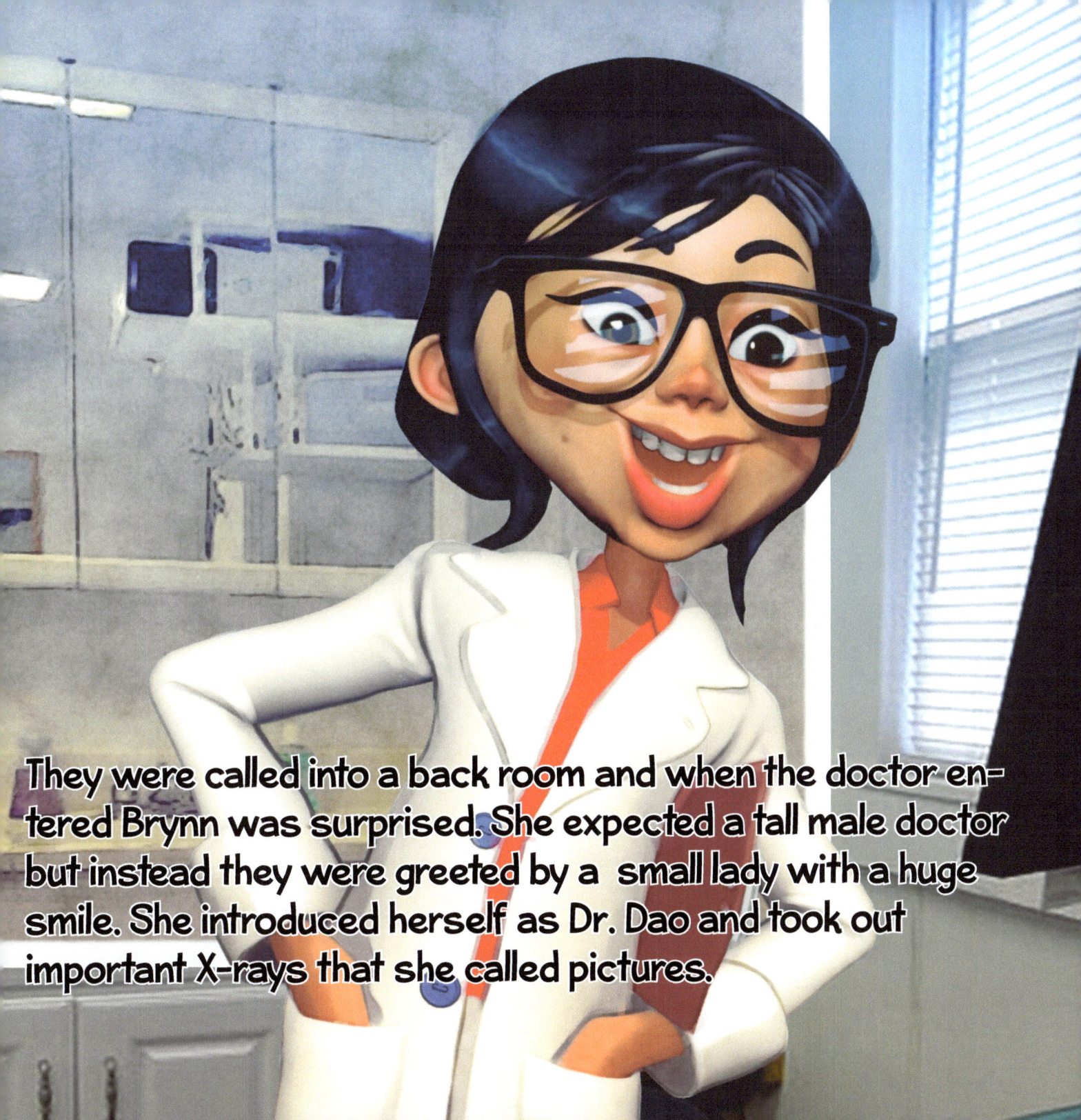

They were called into a back room and when the doctor entered Brynn was surprised. She expected a tall male doctor but instead they were greeted by a small lady with a huge smile. She introduced herself as Dr. Dao and took out important X-rays that she called pictures.

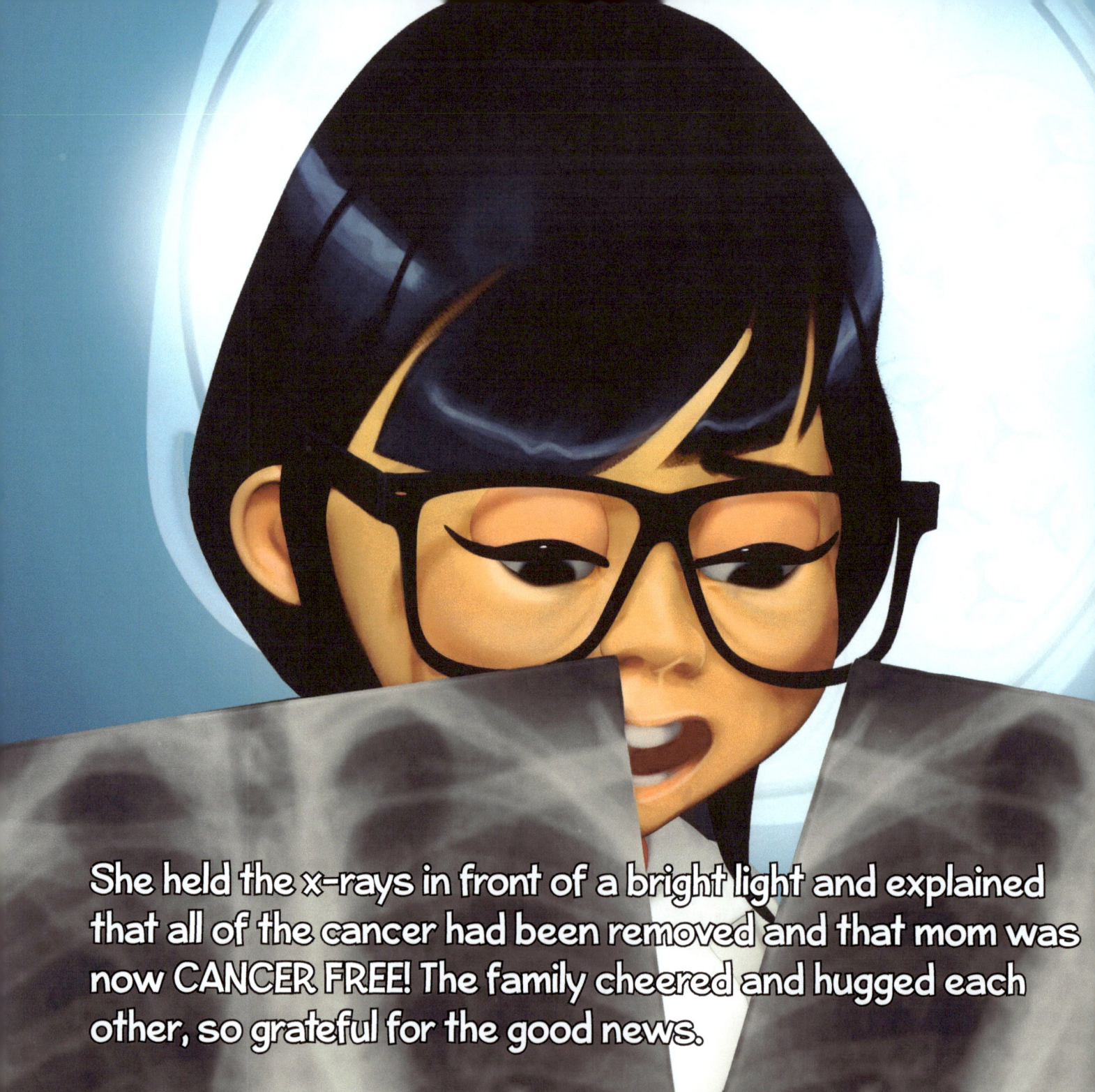

She held the x-rays in front of a bright light and explained that all of the cancer had been removed and that mom was now CANCER FREE! The family cheered and hugged each other, so grateful for the good news.

Before leaving the office, Brynn's mom took her by the hand and said, "Brynn, we are so happy to get the news of my clean bill of health and I want you to know that you played a BIG part of that. You are a brave girl and your courage and hope has helped our family!" "We are sorry you weren't able to have a birthday party and we hope this can make up for it." Then dad handed Brynn an envelope and said,"We know how hard you worked on creating the shirt to show support for mom and how hopeful you feel when you wear it, this is a little gift to help you to get started on creating shirts for other kids with sick parents.

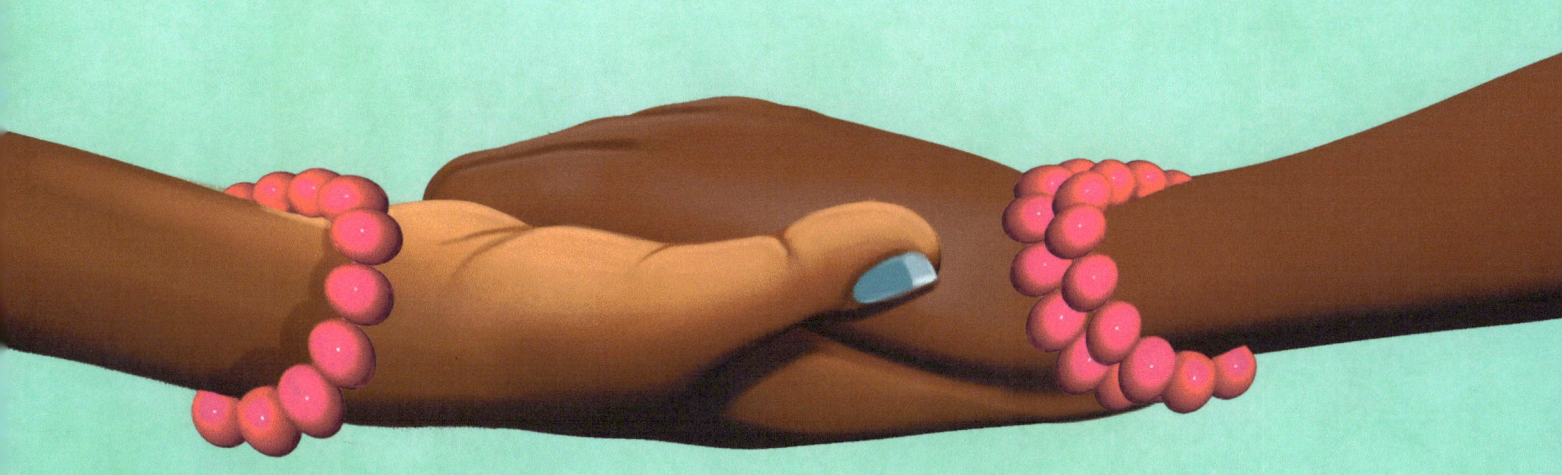

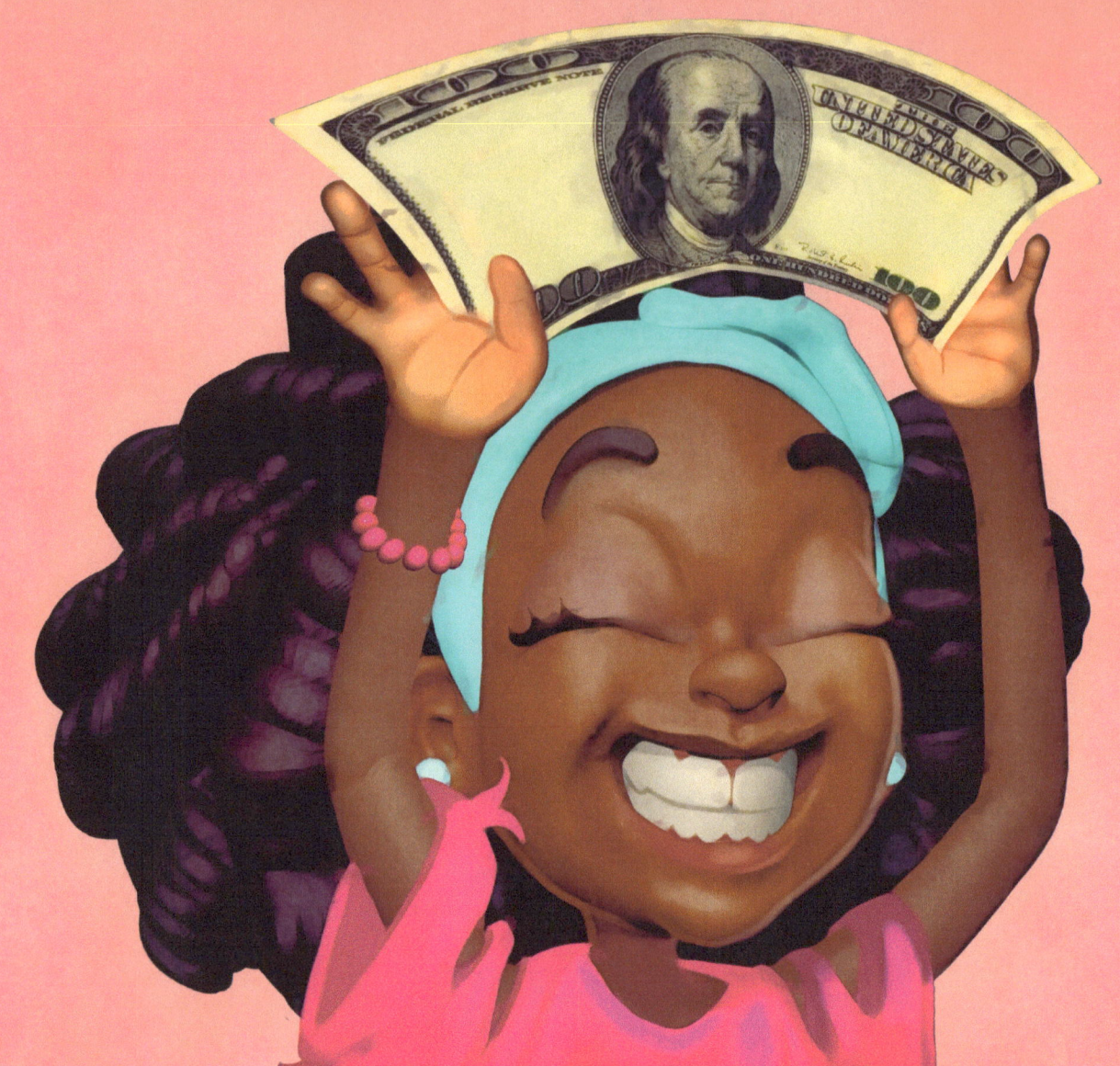

We hope the shirts you create for others, will help them and their parents as much as they've helped our family." When Brynn opened the envelope, a crisp $100 bill fell out. She couldn't help but smile inside.

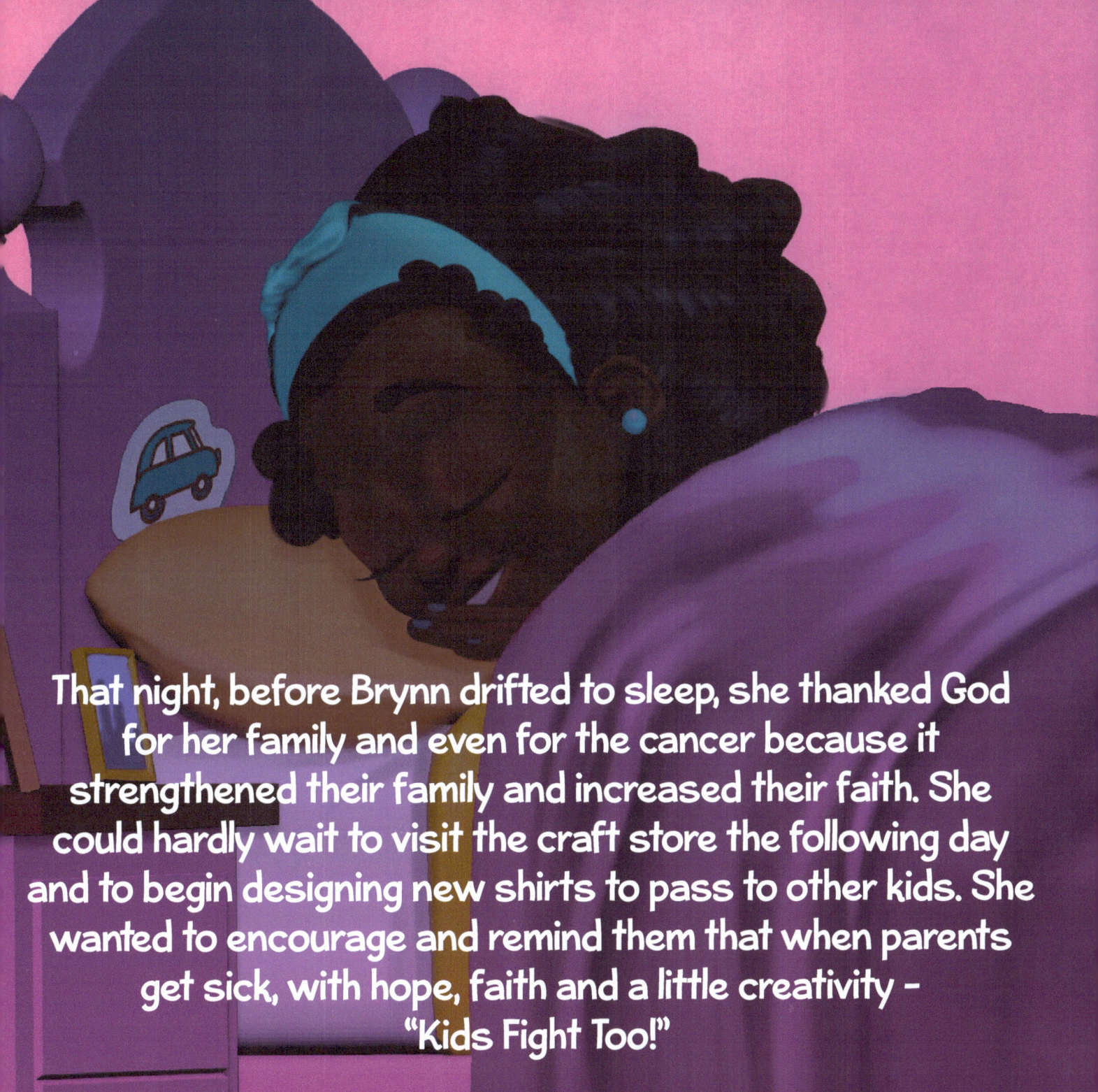

That night, before Brynn drifted to sleep, she thanked God for her family and even for the cancer because it strengthened their family and increased their faith. She could hardly wait to visit the craft store the following day and to begin designing new shirts to pass to other kids. She wanted to encourage and remind them that when parents get sick, with hope, faith and a little creativity –
"Kids Fight Too!"

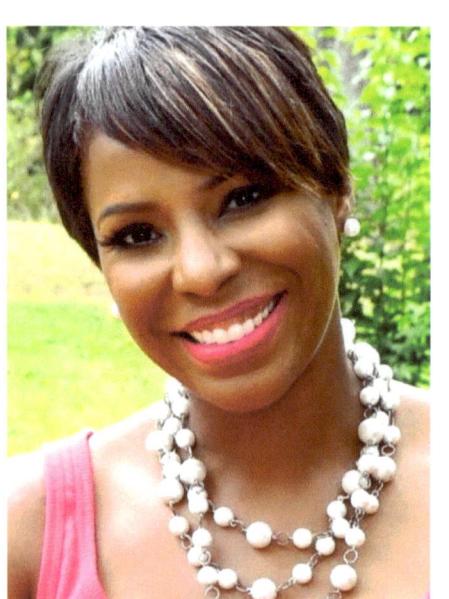

About the Author:

Niki Guinn-Rogers is a wife, mother, educator, counselor and first time children's book author. She is a breast cancer survivor and enjoys sharing her testimony of faith and obedience with others. The idea for this story came when Niki remembered how she was able to draw strength from her own child during her season of sickness. It is her prayer, that Kids Fight Too will help children (and their parents) believe in the power and strength that adults can gain from children during sickness. She hopes to empower children to come up with their own creative ideas during difficult times. She graduated from the University of North Texas with a degree in Human Development & Family Studies and has earned 3 advance degrees. Niki lives in Texas with her husband, Vitto, their 2 kids (Aiden & Hailee) and 2 dogs (Chase & Mya). She enjoys traveling, reading, and making memories with family and friends.

www.nikiguinnrogers.com

nikiguinnrogers@gmail.com

Facebook: Kids Fight Too

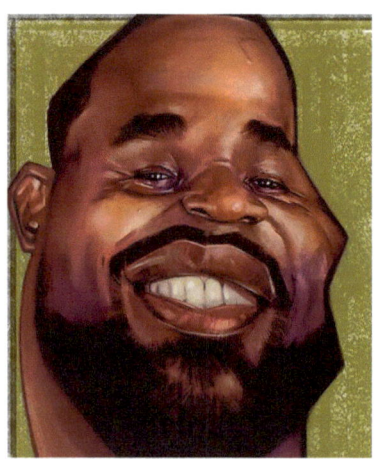

The illustrator

Tyrus Goshay is a digital illustrator and 3d artist with over 16 years of experience. He serves as a college professor, teaching both game design, and illustration in his off time. Tyrus has his bachelors in computer animation and Multimedia, and his masters degree in teaching with technology (malt). He has contributed to several award-winning projects in the world of toy design and has been recognized for his achievements in academia as well. He also has tutorials in illustration and Digital sculpting available for training on the web.
Visit his book store and see other books that he has illustrated.

www.tgosketch.bigcartel.com

Facebook.Com/tgosketch

tgosketch@gmail.com

Instagram/tgosketch